Health Consequences of Service During the Persian Gulf War: Initial Findings and Recommendations for Immediate Action

Committee to Review the Health Consequences of Service
During the Persian Gulf War
Medical Follow-up Agency
Institute of Medicine

NATIONAL ACADEMY PRESS
Washington, D.C. 1995

NATIONAL ACADEMY PRESS 2101 Constitution Avenue, N.W. Washington, D.C. 20418

NOTICE: The project that is the subject of this report was approved by the Governing Board of the National Research Council, whose members are drawn from the councils of the National Academy of Sciences, the National Academy of Engineering, and the Institute of Medicine. The members of the committee responsible for the report were chosen for their special competencies and with regard for appropriate balance.

This report has been reviewed by a group other than the authors according to procedures approved by a Report Review Committee consisting of members of the National Academy of Sciences, the National Academy of Engineering, and the Institute of Medicine.

The Institute of Medicine was chartered in 1970 by the National Academy of Sciences to enlist distinguished members of the appropriate professions in the examination of policy matters pertaining to the health of the public. In this, the Institute acts under both the Academy's 1863 congressional charter responsibility to be an adviser to the federal government and its own initiative in identifying issues of medical care, research, and education. Dr. Kenneth I. Shine is president of the Institute of Medicine.

Support for this study was provided equally by the Department of Veterans Affairs and the Department of Defense (contract no. V101(93)P-1417).

Library of Congress Catalog Card No. 94-74965

International Standard Book No. 0-309-05241-6

Additional copies of the report are available in limited quantities from:
National Academy Press Box 285 2101 Constitution Avenue, N.W. Washington, D.C. 20055
Call 800-624-6242 or 202-334-3313 (in the Washington Metropolitan Area)

B522

Printed in the United States of America

The serpent has been a symbol of long life, healing, and knowledge among almost all cultures and religions since the beginning of recorded history. The image adopted as a logo-type by the Institute of Medicine is based on a relief carving from ancient Greece, now held by the Staatlichemuseen in Berlin.

Committee to Review the Health Consequences of Service During the Persian Gulf War

JOHN C. BAILAR III,* *Chairman,* Professor, Department of Epidemiology and Biostatistics, McGill University Faculty of Medicine, Montreal, Canada

CHRISTOPHER C. GREEN, Director, Technology Research Partnerships, General Motors Corporation, Warren, Michigan

RICHARD B. HORNICK, Vice President of Medical Education, Orlando Regional Healthcare System, Medical Education Administration, Orlando, Florida

KARL T. KELSEY, Associate Professor of Radiobiology and Occupational Medicine, Harvard School of Public Health, Boston, Massachusetts

WAYNE M. LEDNAR, Medical Director, Rochester Medical Services, Eastman Kodak Company, Rochester, New York

THOMAS A. LOUIS, Professor and Head, Division of Biostatistics, University of Minnesota School of Public Health, Minneapolis, Minnesota

GARY M. MARSH, Professor, Department of Biostatistics, University of Pittsburgh Graduate School of Public Health, Pittsburgh, Pennsylvania

DAVID P. RALL,* Institute of Medicine Foreign Secretary, Washington, D.C.

PHILIP K. RUSSELL, Professor, International Health, School of Hygiene and Public Health, Johns Hopkins University, Baltimore, Maryland

DAVID A. SAVITZ, Professor, Department of Epidemiology, School of Public Health, University of North Carolina, Chapel Hill, North Carolina

G. MARIE SWANSON, Professor, Department of Medicine and Director, Cancer Center Michigan State University, East Lansing, Michigan

GUTHRIE L. TURNER, Jr., Chief Medical Consultant, Division of Disability Determination Services, Department of Social and Health Services, Olympia, Washington

MARK J. UTELL, Professor of Medicine and Environmental Medicine, Department of Medicine, Pulmonary and Critical Care Unit, University of Rochester School of Medicine, Rochester, New York

JAMES H. WARE, Dean, Academic Affairs Harvard School of Public Health, Boston, Massachusetts

DAVID H. WEGMAN, Professor and Chair, Department of Work Environment, University of Massachusetts, Lowell, Massachusetts

* Member, Institute of Medicine

LOUIS JOLYON WEST, Professor, Department of Psychiatry and Biobehavioral Sciences, University of California, Los Angeles, School of Medicine, Neuropsychiatric Institute, Los Angeles, California

ELIZABETH WILLIAMS, Department of Internal Medicine, James Quillen College of Medicine, East Tennessee State University, Johnson City, Tennessee

NANCY FUGATE WOODS,* Director, Center for Women's Health Research, Professor, School of Nursing, University of Washington, Seattle, Washington

Study Staff

DIANE J. MUNDT, Study Director and Senior Program Officer
AMANDA E. HULL, Research Assistant
CARLISS PARKER-SMITH, Project Assistant

Preface

The Committee to Review the Health Consequences of Service During the Persian Gulf War was appointed in December 1993 by the Medical Follow-up Agency of the Institute of Medicine (IOM), in response to Public Law 102-585. In response to the IOM role directed in this law, the committee is to provide: "(a) an assessment of the effectiveness of actions taken by the Secretary of Veterans Affairs and the Secretary of Defense to collect and maintain information that is potentially useful for assessing the health consequences of the military service . . . [in the Persian Gulf theater of operations during the Persian Gulf War]; (b) recommendations on means of improving the collection and maintenance of such information; [and] (c) recommendations on whether there is sound scientific basis for an epidemiological study or studies on the health consequences of such service, and if the recommendation is that there is sound scientific basis for such a study or studies, the nature of the study or studies." The joint and equal sponsors of this review, as mandated in the law, are the Department of Veterans Affairs (VA) and the Department of Defense (DoD). The DoD retains responsibility for all medical care of veterans who remain on active duty or retire; the VA is responsible for caring for those who have served in but left the military.

The committee understands that the primary objective in a military operation is to successfully complete the mission, which the DoD accomplished with great distinction in the Persian Gulf. Scientific research is not and cannot be a high priority in the midst of armed conflict. The committee feels that the DoD and VA did and now do a creditable job in addressing the potential health is sues, given the time pressures and public concerns. The committee recognizes that these two agencies experienced various difficulties in meeting the highest scientific standards during the conflict and it is understandable that the results of these gaps still persist, but we believe that some of the most critical problems can still be rectified. This interim report provides constructive criticism of a number of areas that require immediate action.

The task before the IOM committee is expected to take three years; however, there are some matters that could be settled earlier and some findings and recommendations that should be provided immediately because they have implications for ongoing research. This report is the result of the committee's deliberations and conclusions regarding certain issues for which findings are sufficient to make recommendations at this time. The report also includes an overview and some commentary on ongoing activities in the background section of the report. A second, final report should be available by September 1996.

Several topics that the committee has chosen not to include in this first report are on the agenda for further consideration and review for the final report. Among the topics for future consideration are the issues of chronic fatigue syndrome, fibromyalgia, multiple chemical sensitivity, and psychosocial outcomes. Readers should understand that the absence of discussion of some of these topics does not mean that the committee is ignoring them.

Committee members were drawn from several areas of expertise. During our work we have heard from veterans, spouses, and concerned individuals in a public meeting, and through letters, phone calls, and individual contacts. Without prejudging any technical matters, we are impressed by the concern of veterans and their relatives, friends, and organizations about those who are sick and about their dedication to finding the causes of and remedies for the evident human suffering. This concern has deepened as American troops have been deployed to two more distant areas as this report was being finalized.

We hope that this report will be valuable to the VA, DoD and Congress in focusing research in appropriate and effective ways. In the process of writing this report, the committee received valuable assistance from several people who we would like to thank at this time: Ms. Laura Baird, Mr. Michael Edington, and Ms. Rosa Kasper.

JOHN C. BAILAR III, *CHAIR*

Contents

Health Consequences of Service During the Persian Gulf War: Initial Findings and Recommendations for Immediate Action

1

Introduction

This first report by the Institute of Medicine (IOM) Committee to Review Health Consequences of Service during the Persian Gulf War is the result of our review of the current activities related to potential health consequences of service in the Persian Gulf. Our recommendations for actions that should be taken immediately, are the committee's response to concerns by Congress and veterans. In our second report, the committee will focus on reviewing issues requiring additional scientific evaluation, and recommendations will follow from that review.

The IOM committee is issuing these initial findings and recommendations because of the urgent concerns of Persian Gulf War veterans and of society in general, and because some steps can—and should—be taken promptly. The actual scope and nature of the health problems of Persian Gulf veterans have not yet been ascertained. We have not limited our discussions to a narrow interpretation of the charge, but rather have chosen to broaden the scope of our study of health outcomes and related research efforts, to include women's health and reproductive issues, infrastructure and procedures for data collection, health services influences, nutritional problems of military personnel, the role of psychiatric diagnosis, the review of Persian Gulf boards and coordination groups, as well as issues stemming from involvement in the Persian Gulf region that might have relevance to possible future conflicts.

To gather information for this report, committee members listened to invited presentations (see Appendix B), examined the voluminous materials prepared for use by the IOM staff, talked with physicians responsible for treating patients listed in the Department of Veterans Affairs (VA) Persian Gulf War Veterans Health Registry (subsequently referred to in the text as the Persian Gulf Health Registry), and looked at some of their case records. We also talked with other physicians interested in this case material, including one who has helped a few of these patients at her own expense. We have also followed the coverage of unexplained illnesses referred to as the "mystery illness" or "Gulf War Syndrome" (GWS) by the public media.

ORGANIZATION OF THE REPORT

Following the introduction, this report contains two additional chapters. In the second chapter, the committee presents findings and recommendations that should be implemented as soon as possible. Implementing these recommendations is necessary only to enable certain critical research on the health effects associated with service in the Persian Gulf War (PGW), and to establish infrastructure and procedures to support health studies related to possible future military encounters. The chapter is divided into three sections: "Data and Databases," "Coordination/Process," and "Considerations of Study Design Needs." This chapter precedes the supporting background chapter because the committee believes its findings and recommendations are the most important part of the report.

The third chapter provides a general overview and discussion of the actions taken and the steps involved in defining the Persian Gulf health arena. The chapter is divided into the following sections: "Boards and Committees," "Population-Based Activities," "Health-Outcome-Based Activities—Completed or Well Underway," "Health-Outcome-Based Activities—New or Just Beginning," and "Exposure-Based Activities."

Appendix A comprises the putative outcomes and exposures that the committee has been, and will continue to, evaluate and modify as additional information becomes available; Appendix B is a listing of invited presentations; Appendix C contains relevant portions of the laws that are mentioned in this report.

Included in Appendix D are the dates of each IOM committee meeting, a list of persons who presented or submitted testimony for the committee's public meeting, and a list of persons who have subsequently sent materials to the IOM committee.

Appendix E includes a list of activities known to this committee to be related to the Persian Gulf health experience, as of September 1994 and Appendix F includes a timeline of events beginning with the invasion of Kuwait and continuing with events and activities related to this report.

The second report from this committee will build on materials presented here, and will report additional recommendations that may evolve from deliberations on issues that have not been resolved for this report.

HISTORY OF EVENTS IN THE PERSIAN GULF WAR

On August 2, 1990, Saddam Hussein's Iraqi troops invaded Kuwait. In response to this invasion, U.S. Naval forces were strengthened in the area to enforce trade sanctions, and an aircraft carrier with 2,100 Marines was sent to join other carriers in the area. More U.S. ground troops were deployed to Southwest Asia (SWA) theater of operations (Persian Gulf, Iraq, Kuwait, Saudi Arabia. Red Sea, Gulf of Oman, Gulf of Aden, portion of Arabian Sea (northern), Oman, Bahrain, Qatar, and United Arab Emirates), beginning on August 7, 1990. This deployment of troops was known as Operation Desert Shield. By August 22, 1990, the president announced the mobilization of reserve forces, including many Army noncombat personnel.

The build up continued, and on November 8, 1990, President George Bush announced the deployment of additional troops to join the troops already stationed in SWA. On November 29, 1990 the United Nations (UN) Security Council passed Resolution 678, which authorized the UN member states to use "all necessary means" to remove Iraqi troops from Kuwait. On January 12, 1991 Congress passed House Joint Resolution 77, which authorized President Bush to use armed forces in the region to implement UN resolution 678. On January 14, this resolution was signed into law as Public Law (PL) 102-1. On January 16, 1991, the coalition air forces began attacking Iraqi targets. These actions have been termed Operation Desert Storm (ODS).

Oil fires in Kuwait started burning on February 20, 1991. The ground war began on February 24, 1991, as the coalition forces attacked Iraqis in Kuwait and southern Iraq. By February 28, 1991, the war was over, and the last troops to have participated in the ground war returned home on June 13, 1991. The last oil field fire was extinguished by early November 1991. This history of events in the Persian Gulf was condensed from a chronology report to Congress (CRS, 1992).

In all, a total of approximately 700,000 U.S. troops had been deployed to the Persian Gulf theater for Operation Desert Shield/Desert Storm (ODS/S). As troops were being deployed, others were returning home; the maximum number of troops located in the Persian Gulf was in February 1991, with a rapid return of troops after March 1991. The number of reserve and active duty troops located in the theater of operations, by month, is shown in Figure 1. A timeline of these events and subsequent activities relevant to this report is in Appendix F.

Since the earlier days of this operation the U.S. government, and military and civilian personnel assigned to the Persian Gulf, and their families have been concerned about the possible health consequences of serving in the Persian Gulf theater of operations. Following the Persian Gulf War, Congress mandated, through PL 102-190, that the Department of Defense (DoD) establish the Persian Gulf Registry, to determine the location of members of the Armed Forces exposed to burning oil fumes during Operation Desert Storm. Subsequently, in PL 102-585, passed on November 4, 1992, the Persian Gulf Registry mandate to DoD was expanded to include the location of "any other members who served in the Operation Desert Storm theater of operations during the Persian Gulf conflict." Records of the DoD register are designed to include service members' names and other relevant identifying information, the grid location of their service in the Gulf, and the prevailing atmospheric and other environmental conditions, including length of time exposed to burning oil fumes.

In addition, PL 102-585 also mandated that the Department of Veterans Affairs establish a Persian Gulf War Veterans Health Registry, and that it record relevant medical data on members of the Armed Forces who served in the Persian Gulf theater of operations during the Persian Gulf War. This registry contains names and selected other personal and health data, and includes PGW veterans who have sought VA care or medical examination, or who claim disability based on PGW service; active duty service members seeking similar health examinations because of PGW service from DoD medical facilities; and veterans for whom beneficiaries have filed claims (see Appendix C).

PL 102-585 also requires the Secretary of Veterans Affairs and the Secretary of Defense jointly to seek to enter into an agreement with the Medical Follow-up Agency (MFUA) in the Institute of Medicine, in the National Academy of Sciences (NAS), to report on "(a) an assessment of the effectiveness of actions taken by the Secretary of Veterans Affairs and the Secretary of Defense to collect and maintain information that is potentially useful for assessing the health consequences of the military service . . . [in the Persian Gulf theater of operations during the PGW]; (b) recommendations on means of improving the collection and maintenance of such information; [and] (c) recommendations on whether there is sound scientific basis for an epidemiological study or studies on the health consequences of such service, and if the recommendation is that there is sound scientific basis for such a study or studies, the nature of the study or studies" (see Appendix C).

The contract with the IOM was funded jointly by VA and DoD beginning on September 30, 1993. The IOM Committee to Review the Health Consequences of Service during the Persian Gulf War was approved December 31, 1993, by the IOM and National Research Council (NRC), which is the operating arm of the NAS. The efforts of the committee from January 1994 through this writing in September 1994, have focused on reviewing Persian Gulf (PG) related activities to date, and making recommendations based on that review. The process has included five committee meetings prior to the release of this report and a review of numerous documents sent to the committee for consideration. The second meeting, which took place on the afternoon of February 28 and the morning of March 1, 1994, included a public meeting in Washington, D.C. to allow presentations from anyone who wished to address the committee members. Additional written materials received after the public meeting were made available to the committee members to review (see Appendix D).

Although the products of oil well fires were the initial focus of concern about the health effects of the PGW, attention has shifted to a complex of ill-defined and often poorly characterized symptoms and signs of illness. In response to the growing concern about unexplained illnesses, several boards were established by federal government agencies, composed of representatives from VA, DoD, Environmental Protection Agency (EPA), and Department of Health and Human Services (HHS). The VA's Persian Gulf Expert Scientific Committee is reviewing all aspects of patient care, and medical diagnoses, and is providing professional consultation as needed. A DoD Task Force of the Defense Science Board (DSB) reported on the cause and effect of the full range of low-level chemical exposure, environment pollutants, endemic biologics, and other health hazards that might have affected Persian Gulf veterans (DSB, 1994).

The Persian Gulf Veterans Coordinating Board, chaired by the Secretaries of Defense, Veterans Affairs, and Health and Human Services, oversees the coordination of all efforts in research, clinical care and disability determination/ compensation for illness related to service in ODS/S. The Persian Gulf Interagency Research Coordinating Council serves as the research working group of the Persian Gulf Veterans Coordinating Board, which coordinates all Persian Gulf health consequences research activities of the Executive Branch of the Federal Government. In April 1994, the Persian Gulf Interagency Research Coordinating Council sponsored a Technology Assessment Workshop held at the National Institutes of Health (NIH) entitled "The Persian Gulf Experience and Health." This workshop, and the boards mentioned above are discussed in greater detail in chapter 3.

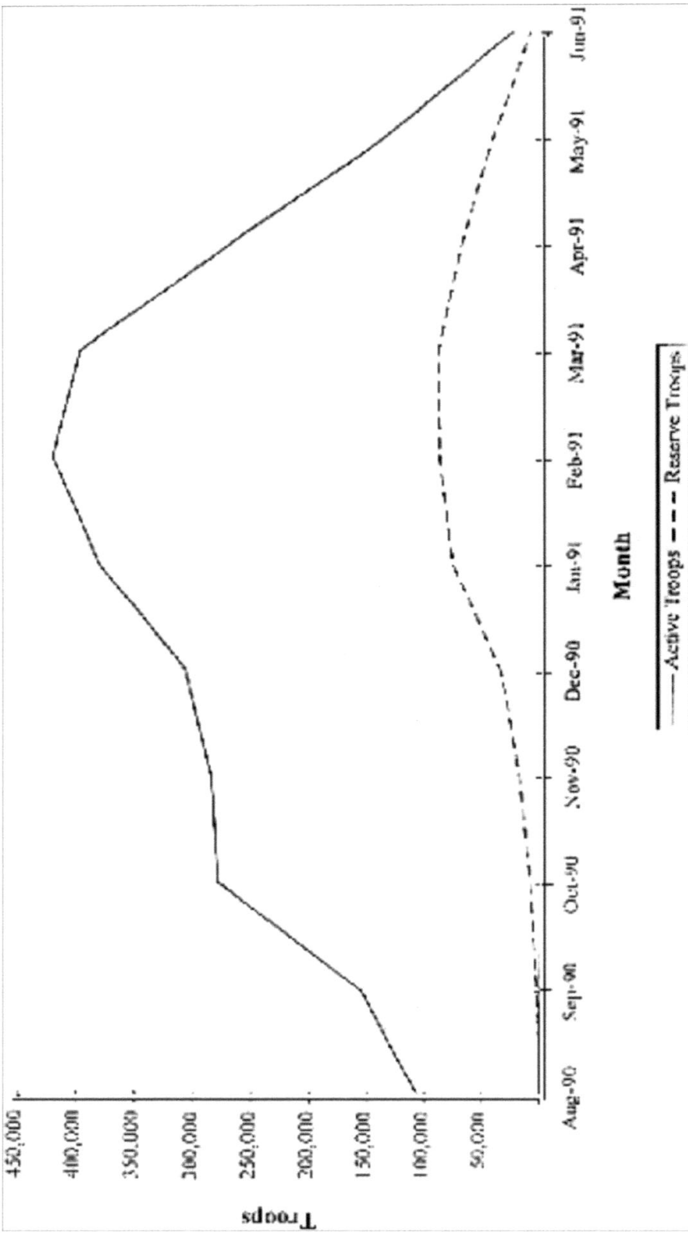

Figure 1. Number of U.S. troops in the Persian Gulf Theater of operations by month.
Source: Information provided by the Defense Manpower Data Center.

2

Findings and Recommendations

In this report, the IOM Committee has attempted to highlight issues we believe would benefit from immediate action. In reviewing the large volume of documents and the progress of research currently underway, we have identified areas that need prompt attention. As the scope and extent of health problems of Persian Gulf veterans have appeared to expand, the social response also has grown. The committee believes that this has resulted in a fragmented attempt to solve these problems. Thus we believe that sustained, coordinated and serious efforts must be made in the near term to focus both the medical, social, and research response of the Government and of individuals and researchers. Hence, the findings and recommendations that follow are offered with the intent to focus and sharpen the debate, and to improve the quality of the data, and thereby, scientific inference. Finally, we hope to impact in a positive way the health in persons who served in the Persian Gulf War, as well as in those who may follow in other military encounters.

Recommendations for immediate action follow based on the findings presented here and the background information presented in the next chapter. The recommendations are to be viewed as independent, and are not presented in any priority order within categories. The recommendations are divided into three categories: data and databases, coordination/process, and considerations of study design needs.

DATA AND DATABASES

Finding 1

The VA Persian Gulf Health Registry is not a population database and is not administered uniformly, therefore, it cannot serve the purposes of research into the etiology or treatment of possible health problems. The Committee recognizes that certain tabulated descriptions of affected persons may legitimately be carried out for reasons other than the generation of scientific data. Specifically, there may be medical reasons for collecting information about patients with certain kinds of problems, especially diagnostic problems, particularly in medical settings where the information may be subjected to more intense scrutiny. An example is the establishment of the VA referral centers for Gulf War veterans. Since a limited number of veterans have been referred to these centers, and because the sample is self-selected, the Committee concludes that it is unlikely that productive scientific research (especially of an epidemiological nature) can ever be based on the data generated by the referral centers or the health registry as currently organized.

Recommendations

- The VA Persian Gulf Health Registry should be limited and specific to gathering information to determine the types of conditions reported. The role of this registry should be clearly defined as a means for identifying and reporting illnesses among Gulf War veterans with concerns about their health. There should be efforts to implement quality control and standardization of data collected by the registry from other VA facilities. The VA registry data should not be promoted or described as a means to determine prevalence estimates or identify the etiology of a disease, but should be reviewed promptly for enrollment trends and potential sentinel events.
- The VA should improve publicity regarding the existence of the Persian Gulf Health Registry, and encourage all concerned PGW veterans to be registered.
- Where possible the referral centers standardized protocol should be used in each VA facility.
- The timeliness of data received from the VA Medical Centers (VAMC) to be entered into the PG Health Registry database needs to be improved.

Finding 2

No single comprehensive data system exists that enables researchers to track the health of Persian Gulf War veterans both while on active duty and after separation. As a result, it is not possible to conduct research and determine the morbidity and mortality experience of this population. Although both the VA and the DoD have medical records systems in place, they are inadequate and unlinked. This lack of a single data system is a hindrance to research concerning delayed health effects, both for Persian Gulf veterans and for those serving in future encounters.

Recommendation

- The Vice President of the United States should chair a committee composed of representatives from HHS, DoD and VA to devise a plan to link data systems on health outcomes with the development of standardized health forms, the ability to access information rapidly, and an organized system of records for rapid entry into the data system.

Finding 3

The characteristics of the population at risk are critical to any definitive studies of Gulf War health effects. The DoD has taken the proper steps to enumerate and describe this population that will be part of the planned, but yet incomplete, Army Geographical Information System model.

Recommendations

- The DoD registry needs to be completed as quickly and accurately as possible.
- The Secretaries of DoD and VA should develop a single service-connected health record, for each present active duty and former service member. All health data entries should be recorded in this single record for the individual.

COORDINATION/PROCESS

Finding 4

The committee has noted with interest and some concern the wide variety of disciplines and expertise among persons who have considered possible causes of a mystery illness. It has appeared to the committee that some of these persons and organizations are simply not qualified to draw reasoned scientific conclusions, or to implement those conclusions by means of specific medical intervention. There may be substantial risk from inappropriate interventions because of adverse reactions to drugs, development of resistant strains of microorganisms, or especially the diversion of attention away from more orthodox diagnoses and treatments that hold some promise of relief from symptoms of a "mystery illness."

Recommendation

- Decisions to provide funding, to refer patients, or to change usual operating procedures for providing financial support should be based on more solid scientific basis than has sometimes been evident in prior resource allocation. Funding should be subject to external peer review and approval.

Finding 5

There are dozens of studies of PGW health effects underway now, and many others are being initiated. Several efforts appear to be redundant, yet there are clearly gaps where research efforts are necessary. In its final report, the IOM Committee will recommend some additional specific research projects.

Presently, the total number of undiagnosed conditions is unknown because the data either are insufficiently understood or available. Data that are available are fragmented, managed by different methods in different agencies, and based on a wide variety of unconnected rationales, from both military and civilian institutions. Many research efforts should, but do not, rely on a common set of data resources. Because so many unanswered questions remain concerning multi-system etiologies that have been proposed to explain undiagnosed signs and symptoms, all future as well as current evaluations must ensure that findings can be reconciled across studies.

Recommendations

- The Persian Gulf Veterans Coordinating Board (chaired by the Secretaries of VA, DoD, HHS) should actively coordinate all studies developed from any new initiatives that receive federal funding, to prevent unnecessary duplication and to assure that high priority recommended studies be conducted. These studies should undergo appropriate external peer review before, during, and after data collection and analysis.
- More staff should be assigned by the Persian Gulf Veterans Coordinating Board in order to monitor, collect, assemble, and make accessible when appropriate all relevant requested emerging data from studies now underway, and make periodic reports to the appropriate federal oversight authority.
- Each new initiative should be evaluated in the context of what it can contribute. That is, each new study should add something of value to the information already being obtained or accumulated.

CONSIDERATIONS OF STUDY DESIGN NEEDS

Finding 6

To date, most studies of PGW veterans have been piecemeal—one military unit here, one collection of volunteers with some problem there, etc. But, some of these studies have several fundamental problems. They are necessarily incomplete, they usually lack proper controls, they are hard to generalize, they are subject to grave statistical problems because of post-hoc hypotheses and multiple comparisons, and where an effect truly exists they tend to have low statistical power to detect a difference. Thus, bits and pieces are not likely to answer any critical questions. The committee recognizes that an initial effort to survey a sample of veterans is underway, but more is needed.

Overall, there has been a broad and serious lack of adequate attention to the design of individual studies, and even more seriously, the scope and organization of an appropriate collection of studies, each focused on the resolution of a specific question. The committee regards this as a grave, though understandable failure. Experts in research design can and should work shoulder to shoulder with experts in the subject matter of each individual study; this is particularly true for work in epidemiology. A broader view of the whole collection of studies, including input from experts in subject matter and in research methods, persons knowledgeable about data sources and medical care systems, and those with general appreciation of public concerns and public policy has been conspicuously lacking. We believe that good studies could be done, but that they will require substantial input from experts in epidemiological methods.

Recommendations

- The VA and DoD should determine the *specific* research questions that need to be answered. Epidemiologic studies should be designed with the objective of answering these questions given the input of experts in epidemiologic research methods and data analysis, along with the input of experts in the subject matter areas to be investigated.
- To obtain data on symptom prevalence, health status, and diagnosed disease, the Secretaries of DoD and VA should collaborate to conduct a population-based survey of persons who served in the PG, and of PG-era service personnel. The study should be designed to allow for adequate comparisons of outcome by sex, service branch, and rank, with oversampling among certain subgroups to allow for analysis. The IOM committee is willing to comment on and assist in the study design. An evaluation of the feasibility and need for a longitudinal study should take place coincident with this national survey.

Finding 7

Initial characterizations of smoke and unburned contaminants from the oil well fires and other sources are not adequate, nor have the data available been reduced to a format usable for drawing conclusions or conducting health studies. Considerable data exist from a wide number of sources, but they have not been compiled or analyzed in any organized or efficient way. For example, lead levels that would cause acute toxicity have been reported; however, questions about the validity of these reports have not been adequately addressed.

Recommendations

- DoD should assemble and organize these data from all sources for evaluation by the IOM committee.
- DoD should conduct a study that simulates exposure in tents heated by diesel fuel, with composition similar to that used in the PG. Fuels and conditions should simulate as closely as possible the conditions that existed in the PG. Exposure to lead and its possible effects should be explored further. The committee reviewed work done indicating that some personnel in the Gulf had lead levels consistent with acute intoxication. Thus in investigating lead expo

sure, special attention should be given to any history of abdominal pain or mental disorders.

Finding 8

As acknowledged by the investigator, the VA study of mortality in the PG veteran population is of insufficient duration to observe a higher rate of death than would be expected from chronic disease outcomes.

Recommendation

- The VA should plan and provide support for its mortality study to continue in the future in order to permit the detection and investigation of long-term mortality from chronic disease.

Finding 9

Although infertility, unrecognized and recognized pregnancy loss, premature delivery, fetal growth retardation, birth defects, and abnormal development are all components of reproductive health, studies and surveillance efforts to date have focused primarily on birth defects, fetal and neonatal deaths, and low birth weight. Adverse reproductive effects can be mediated through males as well as females, so it is important to study exposures of both parents. Information on infertility and miscarriage has not been included in the VA Health Registry efforts. Moreover, data on outcomes are available only from a single cluster study in Mississippi and the Army Surgeon General's preliminary data evaluation. DoD launched recently a study of reproductive health, and the VA and DoD clinical evaluation protocols provide some surveillance of infertility, miscarriage, birth defects, and infant deaths.

The design of scientific studies to address reproductive risk associated with environmental exposures is complex. A variety of endpoints may occur throughout the continuum beginning with fertility, through intra-uterine, peripartum, and neonatal development, and continuing with effects manifested only later in childhood. Additionally, sophisticated expertise is required to document environmental exposures as the etiology for adverse pregnancy experience. There are research groups in some academic and federal settings that could, if deemed appropriate, conduct such complex research.

Recommendations

- VA and DoD should include reproductive outcomes among the array of health endpoints in surveillance programs based on medical records and individual questionnaires. Medical records, such as those to be included in the Seabees reproductive study and the DoD reproductive health study, would be suitable to ascertain stillbirth, low birth weight, preterm delivery, and major birth defects. Questionnaires such as those administered for the VA health registry exam could, in addition, address questions of infertility and clinically recognized miscarriage.
- The Persian Gulf Veterans Coordinating Board should consider specific exposures that are most likely to adversely affect reproductive health of women, men on both, distinguishing between agents that would affect reproductive health only if exposure occurred at or around the time of critical periods during pregnancy versus those that might have effects that would persist after the cessation of exposure. As specific hypotheses linking exposure and reproductive outcomes are identified, studies that are suitable to providing more conclusive results for those associations should be designed.
- The Persian Gulf Veterans Coordinating Board should remain alert but skeptical about cluster studies such as those underway in Mississippi. Studies of this kind may be valuable in suggesting etiologic hypotheses; however, they have little promise for resolving questions about links between experiences in the Persian Gulf and reproductive health. Population-based studies of reproductive health outcomes are essential to resolve questions of effects of Persian Gulf War service.

Finding 10

Women who did not realize that they were pregnant at the time were deployed to the Gulf; others became pregnant during their service in the Gulf. These groups of women may have been exposed to substances potentially hazardous to themselves and to their unborn babies. A study would permit comparisons of birth outcomes and potential adverse health effects on women exposed at different times in their pregnancies.

Recommendation

- The Persian Gulf Veterans Coordinating Board should conduct a study to compare women deployed to the PG who were or who became pregnant at any time during the Persian Gulf War with an appropriate group of other women who were pregnant, but did not serve in the PGW, to evaluate potential adverse health outcomes to the mother or child. This study shouldonly be done if a sufficient number of women can be identified. Effortsshould be made to gather exposure information relevant to serviceat potentially high-risk times during gestation.

Finding 11

The committee has become aware that rosters exist that contain the names of persons vaccinated with anthrax and botulinum toxoid.

Recommendation

• DoD should maintain its lists of those receiving anthrax and botulinum vaccines for the purpose of conducting follow-up studies on these cohorts.

Finding 12

Troops were given packets of pyridostigmine bromide (PB) pills to be taken as a prophylactic to the threat of nerve agent exposure, at the direction of their commanding officer. PB by itself, in recommended doses, is a safe drug. Additionally, DEET (N, N-diethyl-m-toluamide) and permethrin were used by the troops to prevent insect bites. There is some information about the possible long-term toxicity to humans of DEET absorbed through the skin; however there appears to be little or no information about dermal absorption of permethrin from residues left on clothing, bedding or elsewhere. Although permethrin is generally not applied to skin, animal studies have shown that permethrin is transferred from cloth to skin, and subsequently absorbed (NRC, 1994). There is little information about how PB, DEET and permethrin might interact; interactions among these compounds are possible and are inadequately studied.

Recommendation

- Studies are needed to resolve uncertainties about whether PB, DEET, and permethrin have additive or synergistic effects. Unsubstantiated suggestions that they may have chronic neurotoxic effects need to be tested in carefully controlled studies in appropriate animal models. Appropriate laboratory animal studies of interactions between DEET, PB, and permethrin should be conducted.

Finding 13

Reported symptoms suggestive of visceral leishmanial infections include fever, chronic fatigue, malaise, cough, intermittent diarrhea, abdominal pain, weight loss, anemia, lymphadenopathy, and splenomegaly. The committee has considered two aspects of exposure to *L. tropica* and resulting infection with leishmania: the occurrence of either cutaneous or visceral leishmaniasis; and the possibility that some component of the poorly defined illness referred to as "Gulf War Syndrome" may result from leishmania infection.

Leishmaniasis (*L. tropica*) in PGW veterans has been evaluated in some very limited clinical studies, but not in epidemiological studies. The clinical studies suggest that the complex of symptoms in the PGW veterans diagnosed with leishmaniasis differs from what has been described in the literature for other forms of leishmaniasis. A major limitation to further investigation and diagnosis of leishmaniasis is the lack of an informative serologic test or other easy to use screening tests.

Recommendations

- The DoD Joint Technology Coordination Group II has research responsibilities for infectious diseases of military importance and should give high priority to the development of a screening approach to be used under field conditions expected in deployment, and a useful diagnostic test for *L. tropica*. The board also should review the status of leishmania research, with a view toward either drafting a request for proposals for test development, or the structured coordination of existing activities.
- All physicians should be notified to look for symptoms that are consistent with both leishmania infection and those reported as "GWS." Clear instructions for follow-up actions should be widely communicated through the physician community. Veterans of Desert Storm should be notified that if they have symptoms that may suggest viscerotropic leishmaniasis they should bring this possibility to the attention of the staff at any facility where they obtain any health care, whether it is in the VA system or not. The latter may be particularly important due to the potential for long-term survival of leishmania in the host.
- When it becomes feasible, VA, DoD, or both should conduct an epidemiologic and seroepidemiologic study of leishmaniasis in PGW veterans presenting symptoms or conditions and appropriate controls. Special attention should center on a possible relation between leishmaniasis and the "Gulf War Syndrome."

Finding 14

The ecology and epidemiology of *L. tropica* are insufficiently studied. Many important questions remain unanswered concerning host species, vectors, and means of transmission to military personnel. The possible role of dogs as reservoirs of disease and the existence of vectors other than sandflies are questions that have been raised.

Recommendations

- DoD should closely monitor all information regarding ecological and clinical studies of *L. tropica* being conducted in the U.S. and abroad.
- International and U.S. researchers should be queried concerning any advances in diagnostic techniques for identifying *L. tropica.*

3

Background

Since the Persian Gulf War, the VA and DoD have undertaken various activities to address potential health consequences of service in the Persian Gulf theater, including activities involving the cooperation of several federal agencies. At the time of this writing (September 1994), the committee had learned of and evaluated the activities listed in Appendix E.

The committee sought to determine what is currently known about the health status of PGW veterans, and about their opportunities for exposures to various agents present in their environment and through their occupations in the Persian Gulf. We requested, received, and reviewed information from researchers involved in the activities listed in Appendix E. In addition, persons involved in some of these activities presented their work to the IOM committee in January and August 1994 (see Appendix B). The quantity and quality of supporting materials the committee received about the activities varied widely. Initially, the federal government lacked any overall strategy by means of which to evaluate a range of potential health effects. There is a need to develop a strategy that will promote a better capacity for the government to deal with these problems in future situations.

In an attempt to characterize and evaluate the various research activities as a response to the health concerns of PG veterans, the committee offers the comments in this chapter. We derived our findings and recommendations from the background information we present here.

In this chapter we discuss activities completed and underway in four major categories, boards and committees; population-based activities; activities based on health outcomes, both completed or well underway, and new or just beginning; and exposure assessment activities.

BOARDS AND COMMITTEES

The work of this IOM committee, as mentioned in the introduction, was specified under PL 102-585, with the original charge focusing on possible health effects of the oil well fires. Because concerns about adverse health consequences of the PGW have broadened since the law was passed, the IOM committee has considered the full range of potential health effects. Since PL 102-585 was passed in November 1992, the federal government has conducted and sponsored research activities under the auspices of several agencies, including the Department of Veterans Affairs, Department of Defense, Environmental Protection Agency, and Department of Health and Human Services. The earliest research on potential health consequences included some evaluation of the possible occurrence of post-traumatic stress disorder (PTSD) and the development of models to predict cancer risk from airborne products of the oil well fires. Initially, there were few panels, boards, committees, individuals, or councils to oversee, coordinate, direct, supervise, or advise those conducting the various federal activities.

In May 1993, the VA held the first meeting of an informal "blue ribbon panel" of experts in response to a growing concern that PG veterans were experiencing unexplained illnesses. The group was chartered (October 8, 1993) as the Persian Gulf Expert Scientific Committee to advise the VA Assistant Chief Medical Director for Environmental Medicine and Public Health, and subsequently the VA Undersecretary for Health about medical findings affecting Persian Gulf veterans. The committee is charged to review all aspects of patient care and medical diagnoses, and will provide professional consultation as needed. This VA committee may advise on other areas involving research and development, veteran benefits, and training for patients and staff. The newly chartered committee met in February 1994, and again in April and July 1994. This is an ongoing advisory committee, with no set termination date.

The Department of Defense also assembled a group of experts to examine reports of illnesses that could not be diagnosed. As requested by the Undersecretary of Defense in December 1993, a Task Force of the Defense Science Board (DSB) of the DoD was charged to review scientific and medical evidence relating to long-term health effects of exposure to low levels of neurotoxic agents. The Task Force on Persian Gulf War Health Effects of the DSB first met in December 1993. Dr. Joshua Lederberg, the Rockefeller University, chaired the proceedings. Following the first meeting, the Task Force requested that the charge be changed to focus deliberations on the cause and effect of the full range of exposure to low levels of chemicals, and also to environmental pollutants, endemic biologics, and other health hazards that might affect veterans of the Gulf War. An interim report was released March 15, 1994; the final report was released in June 1994 (DSB, 1994). The final report by the DSB task force does not provide evidence for any specific cause-effect relationships between putative exposures and an undefined illness. The medical nature and the cause or causes of GWS remained undefined by the Task Force. However, several hypotheses were considered, including some comparisons between chronic fatigue syndrome (CFS) and GWS. The DSB task force is convinced that GWS is not due to chemical or biological warfare agents. This Task Force has completed its work.

During this same time, as concern about unexplained illness among Persian Gulf veterans continued to grow, the Secretaries of Defense, Veterans Affairs, and Health and Human Services established a Persian Gulf Veterans Coordinating Board on January 21, 1994, to ensure interagency coordination of all efforts, separate and joint, in research, clinical care, and disability determination and compensation for post-Operation Desert Shield/Desert Storm illnesses (PGVCB, 1994). The board released an interim report of activities April 1994, and an updated report in May 1994.

PL 102-585 also requires that the President of the United States designate an appropriate department or agency of the federal government to coordinate all research activities undertaken or funded by the Executive branch on the health consequences of military service in the Persian Gulf theater of operations during the Persian Gulf War (see Appendix C). On August 31, 1993, President William Clinton designated the VA as the lead agency for this effort, which also includes the DoD, HHS, and EPA. This Persian Gulf Interagency Research Coordinating Council serves as the "Research Working Group" of the PG Veterans Coordinating Board mentioned above.

Representatives of the Persian Gulf Interagency Research Coordinating Council sponsored a National Institutes of Health (NIH) Technology Assessment Workshop entitled The Persian Gulf Experience and Health, held April 27–29, 1994 (NIH Technology Assessment Workshop Panel, 1994). The workshop initially was expected to be a Consensus Development Conference on the issue of multiple chemical sensitivities (MCS), which some persons believe is linked to GWS. However, the Director of NIH determined that this issue would not fit the guidelines for Consensus Development, as not enough is known or generally accepted on the issue of MCS. Therefore, he assigned members of his staff to assist the Persian Gulf Interagency Research Coordinating Council in planning an appropriate workshop to evaluate PG-related health issues.

The two-and-a-half-day workshop considered the following four questions: 1) What is the evidence for an increased incidence of unexpected illnesses attributable to service in the Persian Gulf War? 2) If unexpected illnesses have occurred, what are the components of the most practical working case definition (s) based on existing data? 3) If unexpected illnesses have occurred, what are the plausible etiologies and biological explanations for these unexpected illnesses? 4) What future research is necessary?

The panel was unable to develop a definition of the GWS that could be used to determine whether there is an association between exposures (plausible etiologies) and outcomes (otherwise unexplained illnesses). The panel criticized the lack of research and data available to date, and focused its recommendations on the following: 1) a short health questionnaire aimed at all 700,000 people who served in the PGW; 2) a focused hospital/clinical protocol for DoD and VA to use in their research on CFS; 3) designs for cohort and case-control studies of health effects of the Persian Gulf War; 4) a retrospective cohort study of pulmonary function in veterans; 5) retrospective simulation of exposures of possible health interest; 6) research into potential stressors; 7) development of effective responses to diagnosis and treatment of stress-related conditions; 8) planning for prospective data collection; and 9) further research on leishmaniasis, which has been mentioned as a possible cause of illness in PG veterans (NIH Technology Assessment Workshop Panel, 1994).

Reports of a complex of signs and symptoms among PG veterans that could not be attributed to a known diagnosis have led to concerns about a "mystery illness" or "Gulf War Syndrome." Even though these reports remain controversial, veterans, their families, and veteran service organizations have organized support for persons reporting such signs and symptoms. Although the clinical assessment of PG veterans with undefined illnesses has benefited from some coordination of efforts between the VA, DoD, HHS, and EPA, the responses of various branches of the government have not been fully coordinated, and are not organized around clear clinical and scientific goals.

Through its discussions with the various organizations and groups of investigators charged with investigating the health effects of Persian Gulf War service, the IOM Committee has become aware of the very significant barriers to effective coordination of activities among the various government agencies whose participation in such activities will be essential to their success. It has appeared to the committee that the responsibility of these groups has not been translated into effective action and that the impact on epidemiologic research studies appears to be nil. Large numbers of studies that are too small will not provide answers; if actively coordinated, the joint effort may be more effective in approaching a meaningful study size. The current coordination of many of the activities is on paper only. In fact, when several investigators were contacted regarding their work, they were surprised that other federal agencies had been listed as being involved in the coordination of their research. Addition ally, it has appeared to the committee that the term "coordination," means that information is simply shared between federal agencies (VA, 1994), but does not usually mean that efforts are made to reduce duplication of similar research activities. Therefore, the IOM committee believes that the authority of coordinating bodies to implement changes in programs and procedures within each of these agencies must be increased substantially. In particular, the committee believes that the leadership of the Vice President of the United States will be needed to achieve the coordination required for this effort. Given the necessary authority, the Persian Gulf Veterans Coordinating Board and the Persian Gulf Interagency Research Coordinating Council can play an important role in this effort. The Persian Gulf Veterans Coordinating Board, while serving many useful functions, does not appear to be taking the lead in coordinating research activities. This role *should be filled* by some group, somewhere.

Coordinating bodies also can increase the ability of different agencies to link and to establish compatibility among databases. This will require doing detailed work on eligibility criteria, identifying information for individual records, and defining the variables to be linked. Finally, these coordinating bodies can support efforts to synthesize completed studies and to identify gaps in current knowledge.

GENERAL COMMENTS ON STUDY DESIGN

Although addressing public and individual concerns about long-term health effects of service in the Persian Gulf War were prominent in the initial charge to this committee, this issue has been largely displaced in public discussion by the growing concern that veterans and their families already are experiencing a variety of health effects of Gulf War service, including those known collectively as the Gulf War Syndrome. Groups of veterans and their families were the first to focus public attention on the possible adverse health consequences of service in the Persian Gulf. Their concerns have elicited a variety of institutional responses and investigations, as described in subsequent sections of this chapter. Some of these investigations can be characterized as "hot pursuit" or "cluster" studies of groups of apparently affected veterans. Other responses, especially the creation of the VA Persian Gulf Health Registry, represent efforts to identify and provide care to those self-identified as experiencing health problems consequential to Gulf War service. Though these efforts may be seen as responsive to community concerns and may also provide care to those who are ill, the methods used to select participants and collect data make these undertakings intrinsically unsuitable for systematic study of the health effects of the Gulf War.

Because "hot pursuit" studies and the Persian Gulf Health Registry represent samples of self-identified respondents, the data they provide are not representative of the collective experience of the entire cohort of Gulf War veterans. In the absence of data about the population at risk, these studies provide no information about the frequency of specific illnesses or syndromes in that population. Because no control populations are studied, no attributions of health outcomes to Gulf War service or specific exposures can be made. Moreover, although studies of groups of individuals reporting illness sometimes can yield insight about either the characteristics of the illness or the exposures shared by those affected, these early studies of Gulf War veterans have not achieved either of these objectives. Given the level of public concern about health effects of service in the Persian Gulf War, it is vital that future studies of Gulf War veterans be based on more rigorous epidemiological methods.

Defining the population at risk is the priority task in order to assess the health effects of the Gulf War. Therefore, the Department of Defense must complete its Registry of Unit Locations as soon as possible, and also must request a review of that database by scientists competent to assess its sufficiency for future epidemiological investigations. Developing this population registry will create the potential for several investigations that can define the scope of health effects related to Persian Gulf service. First, it will be possible to perform a population-based survey of the current health status of Gulf War veterans. Second, it will be possible to create a cohort of veterans who can be followed to assess long-term health effects. Third, it will provide a context for the conduct of population-based case-control studies of specific illnesses or syndromes. The merits of each of these approaches to further study the health effects of Gulf War service are discussed in subsequent sections. We emphasize, however, that each of these studies will require the creation of a valid population registry. Finally, the committee believes that every proposal to study Gulf War veterans must be subjected to rigorous scientific review and must be evaluated in the context of other research.

POPULATION-BASED ACTIVITIES

The Department of Defense is assembling a "Registry of Unit Locations" as required originally by PL 102-190 and modified by PL 102-585. The committee concludes that the Registry of Unit Locations has the potential to be an essential data source for epidemiological investigation because it will be the single best source of data about service members discovered to date, and because it will attempt to define the entire population at risk. Designed to include basic demographic and personnel data for every member of the military who served in the Gulf War between January 1, 1991, and the withdrawal of the last troops, also to be included is information on the day-by-day location of all troops at the unit level. This database is designed to interface with a similar computer-based registry of oil well fire exposure data such that individual exposure matrices can be developed. This registry will include procedures both to verify which veteran units served in the Gulf War, and to standardize quality control of the database. Nevertheless, not enough information was available to the IOM committee to determine whether the data will be of a quality suitable for research purposes. Accordingly, this committee has considered ways to improve completeness and accuracy in data acquisition and extraction. The usefulness of this registry in studies of possible cause-effect relations will depend heavily on the quality of the exposure data.

HEALTH-OUTCOME-BASED ACTIVITIES-COMPLETED OR WELL UNDERWAY

Constructing a Case Definition

During and since the Persian Gulf War, a proportion of returned American service personnel have reported conditions that they attribute to their assignment to the Arabian peninsula and its environs, including their experiences during and after the military campaign continuum called Operation Desert Shield and Desert Storm. Most of these medical problems have been diagnosed and treated in the usual way. However some have been misdiagnosed, have defied diagnosis, or have failed to respond to treatment as expected. Of these, some began in the theater of operations before, during, or after the brief period of combat; others followed the service member's return to the U.S., after a time that ranged from days to many months or even years. Furthermore, some of these men and women subsequently became parents, and some of their offspring have suffered birth defects or other ailments.

Over time the symptoms of these persons (some still on active duty, but most returned to civilian life) became increasingly publicized. Networking of various types, inquiries and reports by the media, and responses by politicians to complaints from constituents have coalesced into a broad public perception that there is or may be some type of "mystery illness" resulting from service in the Persian Gulf. Manifestations have been varied from person to person, but often include arthralgia, weakness, fatigue, headache, memory loss, and other mental impairment. Skin rashes and hair loss have also been mentioned frequently. Problems reported in offspring ranged from miscarriage to Down's syndrome to failure to thrive.

No known etiology could account for this collective picture, although descriptive diagnoses could be used for general symptoms (such as alopecia areata versus toxic alopecia versus male-pattern baldness; or adjustment reaction versus neurotic depression versus post-traumatic stress disorder versus malingering). Several hard-to-verify or obscure diseases have been invoked as causes of these reported symptoms, ranging from leishmaniasis to oxidative phosphorylation disorder. The very legitimacy of some mentioned causes has been questioned, such as multiple chemical sensitivity disorder. A variety of toxins have been suspected, including agents of chemical and biological warfare, fumes of both leaded and unleaded fuels, components of smoke from burning oil wells, illicit substitutes for alcohol, and recreational drugs.

Differences in reported rates of the "mystery illness" among different population segments appear to be both substantial and unexplained. For example, there appears to be no similar condition in the indigenous population, which must have been exposed to local environmental hazards, including products of the oil fires, earlier more intensively, and later than the U.S. military forces (Blanck, 1994; DSB, 1994). Similarly, there seems to be no corresponding problem with the "mystery illness" in members of the Allied Armed Forces. At this time, data are not adequate to determine whether substantial differences exist between men and women, regular and reserve troops, and officers and enlisted personnel. These matters also must be considered in framing research questions.

Mystery illnesses are observed from time to time in every population. Approximately 700,000 U.S. military personnel served in the Persian Gulf. Study of a random sample of that number of persons from the U.S. population, of similar age and sex distribution and similar good health at the start of a period of observation, surely would show that some proportion of them would become ill with some kind of "mystery illness" that causes considerable distress and that has not been fully explained and understood within the U.S. medical system. The question thus is not whether there are any "mystery illnesses" among the returning service personnel, but whether the number or characteristics of such conditions exceeds what one might expect if the same persons had not served in the Gulf War. In short, it is not enough to point to a small number of fully confirmed "mystery illnesses;" a control population is needed to provide U.S.-based background rates of such conditions.

Unusual psychological stress has been promoted as a possible cause or contributing factor to the "mystery illness," but there appears to have been no direct comparison of levels of stress with stress levels reported in other conflicts, such as those in Vietnam, Korea, and World War II. The committee notes that many of the military personnel in the Gulf were older reservists, not new recruits. On the other hand, the committee has heard from several secondary sources that persons in the regular military services do not want to complain about health problems that are less than intolerable, because of possible adverse repercussions on their military careers.

One of the major obstacles to doing studies of unexplained illnesses is the lack of a case definition. Several attempts have been made to form such a definition for the purposes of identifying people to include in an epidemiological study.

The committee agrees with the report of the NIH panel that "it is impossible at this time to establish a single case definition" (NIH Technology Assessment Workshop Panel, 1994). The Gulf War illness phenomenon may prove to be a mixture of several illnesses, or may prove not to be associated with a specific exposure or disease. Without understanding the nature and etiology of the phenomenon, investigators must be prepared to adapt their case definition to new information as it emerges.

Still, a provisional case definition is required for certain types of scientific research. For example, a provisional case definition could provide a basis for a case-control study comparing the Gulf War experience of veterans with symptoms meeting the case criterion with veterans without such symptoms. If such a study is undertaken, it should meet usual standards for size, rigor, and clarity of purpose as case-control studies conducted in other settings. In particular, a study should be large enough to identify patterns of exposure or Gulf War experience among those complaining of Gulf War illness.

A provisional case definition also may have a role in clinical management of Gulf War veterans. Such a definition might be used to identify veterans eligible for care for these symptoms at VA hospitals. It should be recognized, however, that any such case definition would not have a firm scientific basis. We concur in the recommendations of the NIH panel that eligibility for medical care not be based on case definition.

The proposals for a case definition developed to date have several elements in common, including service in the Persian Gulf theater (proposed to be the time span of August 8, 1990, to late July 1991 (Sanford, 1994)); a requirement that the person report a combination of several symptoms from a list that includes fatigue; arthralgia; headache; diarrhea; neuropsychiatric complaints (forgetfulness, difficulty concentrating, depression, memory loss, irritability); difficulty sleeping; fever; weight loss; dyspnea; rash; and myalgia; and that the diagnosis be made only when known clinical conditions with similar symptoms have been excluded.

Case definition is, at the moment, handicapped by the lack of any generally recognized pathognomonic physical signs or laboratory findings, and by uncertainty about whether a specific syndrome exists and, if it does exist, its prevalence among Gulf War veterans. The subjectivity of many of the complaints associated with the Gulf War illness creates serious problems for those seeking to investigate the validity and origins of the illness. The symptoms have been widely publicized, and any attempt to estimate the prevalence of the problem from self-reports could be contaminated by well-known problems of self-reporting. Restrictive policies regarding treatment at VA hospitals could create incentives for veterans to report symptoms now as insurance against a future need to seek medical care.

Outbreak Investigations

In response to reports of outbreaks of unexplained signs and symptoms in Gulf War veterans, the DoD conducted two outbreak investigations to determine whether further study of these groups was necessary, or whether these particular "clusters" showed any indicators of common exposures that could be pursued as a connection to the presenting signs and symptoms.

These "hot pursuit" studies, in which investigators focused on reported clusters of symptoms or illnesses among Persian Gulf War veterans, are similar in many respects to the frequent "cluster studies" of illness in the United States with a possible environmental cause (Caldwell, 1990). This analogy is instructive, because many of the investigators who have participated in such cluster studies have become skeptical about their scientific value (Rothman, 1990).

The typical cluster study is characterized by small sample size, an implicit multiple comparisons problem (in that many other groups of people could have been studied but were not, because the individuals did not report a cluster), a poorly identified exposure, and a significant potential for information bias resulting from respondent awareness of the underlying concern. In the environmental domain, these studies rarely have been fruitful (Cutler et al., 1986; Bender et al., 1990). A few of these studies, especially if they are done well, can be useful at the early stages of an investigation by helping to define the problem and by ruling out both some statistical flukes that have been misinterpreted and some possible etiologies. That phase of research on the reported "Gulf War Syndrome" has been completed. The exploratory studies failed to generate useful leads about either the condition or the exposures that might cause it. Proposals for future studies of this type should be scrutinized very carefully. Additional studies of this type are unlikely to be useful, and they may divert attention and resources away from studies that could be useful.

The first "hot pursuit" investigation was reported by Major Robert F. DeFraites, MC, and colleagues (DeFraites et al., 1992) who investigated reports of symptomatic complaints among reservists belonging to the 123d Army Reserve Command (ARCOM), Lafayette, Indiana. Early in 1992, staff of the 123d ARCOM Surgeon's Office became aware of these complaints, which were subsequently reported by members of the 417th Quartermaster Company, Scottsburg, Indiana.

In response to growing concern about these complaints, Major DeFraites visited Fort Benjamin Harrison and neighboring facilities in April 1992. During this visit, 79 reservists were evaluated. All 79 study participants completed a medical questionnaire, and 78 were interviewed using a short symptom inventory. Each reservist interviewed completed a brief psychiatric intake-type interview, and had vital signs measured. All but one of the reservists received a dental examination. All 78 who participated in the interviews also had blood drawn for complete blood count, white blood cell differential, platelet count, erythrocyte sedimentation rate, and liver function studies. All sera were tested for antibody to *Leishmania tropica*. Sera from selected individuals were tested for antibody for brucellosis. Limited comparative data were available from other groups of veterans.

Fatigue was the most common symptom (70 percent). Other systemic symptoms, including fever, abdominal pain, and diarrhea were much less common. The onset of fatigue and associated symptoms tended to occur after redeployment from SWA, except that the onset of diarrhea was more frequent during deployment. No cases of leishmaniasis, brucellosis, or Lyme disease were detected. The objective findings did not suggest a common pattern of illness among the study group members.

Review of potential exposures during ODS/S provided no evidence that the respondents had been exposed to microwaves, chemicals, radiation, or any other environmental hazard. These reservists did report high levels of stress, which may explain some of the symptoms. The investigators noted that the rapid deployment and subsequent redeployment was stressful for many reservists and their families. The investigators believed, however, that PTSD was present in few, if any, of these reservists. The investigators concluded that this study provided no objective evidence of an outbreak of any disease in this group. They thought that the documentable medical problems and illnesses found were typical of a general population with similar demographic characteristics.

When it is not possible to define a population at risk, as in this case, the investigation does not provide a statistical basis for determining whether rates of symptoms or illnesses depart from expected rates by more than ordinary chance variation. Because of the need to contend with the operations of chance, "hot pursuit" is most effective when it focuses on a cluster of a typically rare disease, or when it uncovers a common pattern of exposure. Thus, as noted above, a "hot pursuit" investigation, in which a small group of apparent cases of disease are studied intensely, can on rare occasions be very useful, but it has important limitations. The problem here is that the group coming to clinical evaluation is a small subset of a larger deployed force, and its representativeness to the larger deployed unit is unclear.

As the investigators noted, this study did not use a consistent definition for a "case" of disease. Also, no evidence for a common exposure was found. Because outbreak investigations are not designed to determine rates of symptoms or disease, or to make comparisons to expected population rates, the investigators were able only to conclude that their findings did not appear to be different for such common problems reported as would be found in the general population.

Although DeFraites et al. included their questionnaires and other research instruments as appendices to their report, it is not clear whether and how these instruments were based on standardized questionnaires, nor is the quality of the laboratory measurements documented. Detection limits, sensitivity, and specificity data of tests used (some of which are quite uncommon in the civilian community hospital setting) are not provided. Thus, the interpretation of these laboratory data is necessarily uncertain. This investigation was aided by the use of trained clinical investigators knowledgeable in dental and in psychiatric issues, in particular. This resulted in more precise clinical descriptions in these two important categories and endpoints.

DeFraites et al. reported that symptoms and objective findings seemed to appear in two peaks, one coincident with return from the Gulf, and another some 6 to 8 months after return. They could find no calendar month associations, clustering by activities, or evidence of "dose-response" relationship with increasing length of time in country, which suggests that at least some of the reported symptoms may be related to the reentry of these reservists. The largest proportion of illnesses that caused time lost from work was attributed to injuries, and thus was recognized and explained. The morbidity assessments reported in this investigation do not include data collected by community (civilian) providers, so that only a portion of the health records are available for an unknown subset of participants.

The absence of demonstrable associations between specific symptoms and reported exposures and activities may reflect a limited ability to detect such associations. The similarity of complaints to those observed in civilian (nondeployed) populations may identify either a similarity of the experiences of deployed groups and their civilian peers or reflect a combination of symptoms consistent with complaints in these same persons prior to their activation. Subsets of the deployed may be "hyper-susceptible," on either a biological or an immunological basis or both if exposed or in adjusting to the stresses of this very disruptive, potentially life-threatening activation to military duty.

This study is useful in documenting the absence of a common underlying malady or environmental exposure among a group of reservists who initially appeared to have similar medical problems. It also shows that the complaints of this group did not represent a common pattern of illness or environmental exposure.

Because of the relatively small number of people studied, the absence of a defined population at risk, and the absence of a control group, this study does not rule out more subtle patterns of illness or exposure among the soldiers participating in ODS/S. Nor does the study address the possibility of increased risk for diseases with long latency periods. Somewhat reassuring, however, is that this one study of aspects of a Gulf War-related illness did not show alarming patterns of disease or exposure, other than the possible impact of stress on the troops.

The second "hot pursuit" investigation reported by the DoD involved the Reserve Naval Mobile Construction Battalion 24 (Seabees) (Berg, 1994). Many members of this unit complained of symptoms that they believed were related to their service in SWA. The Asheville, North Carolina detachment was revisited with follow-up questionnaires, personal interviews, and efforts to verify medical diagnoses by reservist-consented contact with medical providers in the community.

A medical team visited the unit in November 1993 to evaluate those Seabees who believed that they were affected. Eighty questionnaires were administered, and the team interviewed Seabees who had been diagnosed as having a medical problem since returning to the United States. Diagnoses were verified by medical record review and by interviews of medical care providers. A special one-page, anonymous questionnaire was administered to veterans, reservists who were not deployed, and a few spouses and significant others.

Respondents included 61 of the 64 members who had served in ODS/S in SWA, and 19 other veterans. The general characteristics of the veterans were unremarkable.

The report centers on the evaluations of the 61 veterans of ODS/S. These veterans reported a variety of symptoms, including fatigue, joint pains, and sleeping problems, but the symptoms did not point to a common underlying medical diagnosis. This study did not identify patterns of disease or exposure that seem to be useful leads for further research.

The number or percentage with verified diagnoses of psychiatric origin was higher than that reported in other deployed units surveyed to date. Those without verified diagnoses had considerably shorter (presumably milder) illnesses with minimal lost time.

The report included self-evaluation of whether specific symptoms were worse, the same, better, or gone in the past year. These reports are helpful to determine which conditions appear to be self-limiting. The symptoms with the greatest "worsening" (joint pains, fatigue, and confusion) may be useful in defining symptom clusters for additional investigation. Symptoms with the most improvement (diarrhea, rash, sleeping problems, and depression) may reflect infections originating in the Persian Gulf that are self-limited and mild or adjustment reactions that have been resolved. Exposure data in the study were nonspecific and of questionable value. Sera were not banked in this investigation; however, subsequent recommendations from the Navy indicated that banked sera may be useful after diagnostic categories and etiologies of interest are identified.

This study should be viewed as a simple cluster study of 61 Gulf War veterans in a unit that reported an unusual number of health complaints. Much of the report is devoted to comparisons between the veterans with and without a diagnosis found in the DSM-III (APA, 1987), but this comparison is of little value. Like the study of DeFraites et al., this study does not identify either a pattern of illness or a pattern of exposures that would potentially explain the Gulf War syndrome.

Given the information that these first two rounds of investigation provided, further study of this cluster is not likely to be useful.

VA Health Registry and Clinical Evaluations

PL 102-585 included an instruction to the Secretary of Veterans Affairs to establish and maintain a Persian Gulf Health Registry; the purpose and nature of the registry were not specified. The committee has reviewed the systems that have been put into place to collect data relevant to the follow-up of Gulf War veterans. Major ongoing efforts include the PG Family Support Centers, the Persian Gulf Health Registry Examination ("Health Registry Exam"), and the three PG referral centers.

The committee concludes that the Persian Gulf Health Registry may be a valuable clinical tool, but it does not provide information on etiology or disease frequency, and cannot be used alone for research on these matters.

The Health Registry Exam has been used in attempts to standardize both the clinical approach to the Persian Gulf veteran with health problems, and to standardize clinical data collection. The registry data are computerized; however, there appears to be a considerable lag in time between data collection and entry into the computer database. The Health Registry may help to encourage uniform treatment of some of the ailments related to the Gulf War and make it easier to identify cases of illness that could be regarded as sentinel events. It also will further focus the VA on the directed care of Gulf War veterans. The committee has discussed particulars of the examination and data collection (including data quality), and has found that improvements are feasible and needed.

The committee also is concerned about the desire for the Health Registry to go beyond the provision of clinical data. At present, this Health Registry includes data only on veterans who volunteer for evaluation, and so it cannot be used to estimate the frequency of health problems in Gulf War veterans, or to derive unbiased information on disease-exposure associations. Hence, this Registry cannot be used in the epidemiological evaluation of possible associations between service in the Gulf War and important disease outcomes.

Some patients seen for Registry examinations in a VAMC have unexplained illnesses. If a PG veteran has unusual symptoms that cannot be diagnosed or managed at the local VAMC, the patient is referred to one of three special referral centers located at VA medical centers in Washington, D.C., Houston, Texas, and West Los Angeles, California. Patients referred from local VAMCs to one of these referral centers are followed with consultation and referral back to the local VAMC. These centers were selected, according to the VA, on the basis of the availability of clinical and academic expertise in such areas as pulmonary and infectious diseases, immunology, neuropsychology, and toxicology (VA, 1992a). The clinical assessments at these three centers were not standardized until recently (Farrar, 1994). This clinical protocol has been shared with the Department of Defense researchers and it is the basis for their clinical assessments in the Comprehensive Clinical Evaluation Program (CCEP). The Assistant Secretary of Defense for Health has initiated a program of standard assessments for Gulf War veterans who are still in active military status. Information from this activity should be combined with that from the VA study, so that for clinical uses each study could take advantage of the other regarding the assessment. However, for reasons already noted including reports that active duty personnel may not report symptoms because of their fear of medical discharge, even a combined data set is unlikely to be useful for research.

Given the wide variation in reporting of numbers of veterans who claim to be ill with undiagnosed signs and symptoms, and the fact that the combined total of referrals to these three centers to date is approximately 140 (August 1994), it seems that large numbers of veterans with complaints have not been seen for clinical examinations in these centers. This committee does not know whether this discrepancy is because veterans are unaware of their right to a registry exam, because information has not been adequately disseminated, or because the number of undiagnosed ill veterans is not as large as publicized.

Mental Health

The committee notes that the open, direct conflict in the Gulf was very brief—approximately 100 hours—though persons far from the front lines were vulnerable to certain kinds of airborne attacks over a much longer time. In-theater casualties everywhere were quite low for an armed conflict, and the war was seen from its opening moments as being highly successful. The committee has no way to directly compare levels of stress with those in other conflicts, but we believe that the total long-term level of stress among military personnel in the Gulf may well have been substantially lower than the average levels of stress among troops of other wars. However, the stresses of the Persian Gulf may not have been the "usual" combat stresses of war, though they were no less real to the persons affected.

The incidence of PTSD, both acute and chronic, in a given population will depend on a host of variables, including the severity and nature of the stressor(s) experienced by each person; predisposing factors ranging from genetic and developmental to preparatory training and interpersonal support networks, or their absence; comorbidity—both physical and psychiatric—timing and effectiveness of initial treatment; and subsequent experiences. It is not surprising that some Gulf War veterans developed manifestations of PTSD, either immediate or delayed (that is, onset more than six months after the stressful experience). From an understanding of PTSD in other settings, one would expect a higher incidence among reserves than among regular troops, because of factors related to selection criteria, nature of training, likelihood of prior combat experience and command structure differences between these two groups. Physical illness can be a predisposing factor, but it also can coexist with PTSD; so that a diagnosis of PTSD does not eliminate the possibility of an organic illness, obvious or subtle.

Not all psychiatric reactions to environmental stress are classifiable as PTSD. A stressor that generates a classic case of PTSD in one person may produce a monosymptomatic neurosis in one of his or her comrades, a psychotic break in a second, a behavioral aberration in a third, and no apparent pathology in a half-dozen others. The caveat about comorbidity, mentioned above for PTSD, also applies to all of these. Finally, there is an expected incidence of many different psychiatric disorders in any given population; therefore, without appropriate controls we could not even approach a conclusion. Veterans hospitals around the United States have completed several formal and informal psychological studies of veterans returning after the Persian Gulf War. Primarily, these studies were convenience samples not determined scientifically, and had variable rates of participation and completion. Although these studies were essentially descriptive, conducted in many settings, and variable in methods used, the results showed fairly consistent findings, and indications of positive results. The IOM committee received information on some of these individual studies as well as a preliminary report summarizing VA experience with troops experiencing war-related stress (VA, 1992b). The studies were conducted in response to PL 102-25, which required an assessment of the needs for rehabilitative services among PG returnees who experience PTSD, programs and resources available to meet those needs, current plans for providing services, the need for additional resources, and plans to coordinate treatment efforts with the DoD.

These studies indicate that the prevalence of diagnosed PTSD was low among returning veterans, but substantial numbers of veterans appear to have experienced a variety of adjustment problems, and many soldiers may have found their problems highly stressful. It seems likely that post-deployment stress contributed to the health problems some soldiers experienced.

Although the findings strongly indicate the occurrence of PTSD, they make no claim of providing a definitive estimated value. These problems were frequently described as related to work or family. Because most of these studies either recruited volunteers or persons who appeared for medical or mental health evaluations, they do not provide accurate estimates of the prevalence of these disorders among Persian Gulf veterans. In addition, although the use of multiple diverse measures may help to validate observations obtained in several ways, the lack of coordination in the effort (for example, not using a core package of instruments) contributes to the difficulty in estimating the prevalence of problems.

The Fort Devens Reunion Survey, Boston VA Medical Center, was one of the earliest efforts to collect empirical data on returning military personnel following the conclusion of Operation Desert Storm. Phase I was a study of returning military personnel that examined behavioral and psychological impacts of war zone experiences. The study population was drawn from 84 units that returned through Fort Devens, Massachusetts, including National Guard (64 percent), reservists (25 percent), and active duty (11 percent). All participants were surveyed within 5 days of arrival at Fort Devens through a self-reported questionnaire. Included were a number of previously validated measures of psychological distress and PTSD symptomatology. The findings were evaluated with respect to race, sex, service status, and stressor exposure determined by questions related to perceived stressors and 3 other surveys. Only 30 percent of those surveyed had more than minimal level of combat exposure. The survey results are largely descriptive with low frequencies of PTSD scores (9 percent women, 4 percent men) and frequencies of general psychological distress reported (approximately 30 percent of both sexes) (VA, 1992b). The Phase I survey has provided good baseline data against which trends and other changes over time can be measured.

Weaknesses of the study are as follows: 1) some attempt should be made to link the data in Phase I of the Reunion Survey to data that will be generated from the DoD exposure databases in order to assess possible exposure-response relationships; and 2) the 84-unit study population is not a random sample, nor is it necessarily representative of the troops that served in the PGW. Therefore, inferences drawn from this survey cannot be extended with confidence to the total study population of PGW veterans.

To provide data on changes associated with readjustment during the first year of return from the PGW, a Phase II survey was planned for a year after

Phase I. The Phase II survey will provide critical data on the course and possible persistence of the patterns noted in Phase I. Similarly, the follow-up data will elucidate conditions that may have delayed symptom onset. Phase II also will offer data on the longitudinal course of readjustment, and on important subsets of the veteran population. Some findings from Phase II have been completed (Wolfe et al., 1993). Phase III involves an evaluation of cognitive function in a subset (150 to 200) selected from the larger Fort Devens cohort. These people are being evaluated at the Boston VA Medical Center. The study is underway.

In the other studies in which first year findings were reported (VA, 1992b), the prevalence of PTSD is between 4 percent and 16 percent of returnees, depending on demographics and war-zone exposure; women appear to be more prone to PTSD than do men. Studies document the major stressors (including less obvious ones like "waiting around"). These are good studies of a focused endpoint over a short time period. They document well the possible problems with the data and the analysis (for example, nonresponse and selected samples), apply validated psychometric scales, and make an attempt to include a broad group within each of their "catchment" pools.

The Department of Military Psychiatry, Walter Reed Army Institute of Research (WRAIR), Washington, D.C. provided the IOM committee with extensive information. Concern about the psychological stress that would be created by the high-threat deployment to a harsh environment prompted senior Army leaders to learn more about the stress of the deployment. A research team was sent to SWA to study the deployment from September 20, 1990, to October 6, 1990. More than 500 deployed soldiers ranging from privates to lieutenant generals took part in semistructured interviews either as individuals or in small groups of those of similar rank without their supervisors present. Units that had been in SWA longest, were most forward deployed, lived under the most austere conditions, or had missions judged particularly stressful by higher headquarters were studied. At the time of the interviews, small-unit cohesion was high and morale was generally good. Problems in morale or cohesion generally were traceable to factors existing before the deployment, such as deficiencies in trust or communication up and down the chain of command (Marlowe et al., 1990).

This was a broadly focused program designed to evaluate stress and adaptation in ODS/S and to study it both in the context of community and as factors particular to individuals. Assessments of stressors, adaptation, cohesion, morale, and several indicators of mental health were completed before the air and ground war began in SWA, during combat, and following redeployment. These assessments demonstrate a wide range of military-related and nonmilitary-related (family) stressors, and differences between the wartime experiences of active duty service members and reservists. Peak stresses occurred prior to the ground war, with acute stresses of combat being different in nature. Compared with statistics from Vietnam-era veterans, the estimated risk of PTSD was low, about 3 to 4 percent. Several factors, military and nonmilitary, are suggested as mediating the effects of combat stress on outcome, including immediate debriefing, good leadership in the field, and family contact.

Leishmaniasis

An exposure of concern to the troops in SWA was the bite of the sandfly, which may have carried the parasite that causes leishmaniasis. Usually, visceral leishmaniasis is caused by *L. donovani*, *L. chagasi* or *L. infantum*, but exposures during Desert Storm were to *L. tropica*, making the diagnosis more difficult. The committee has considered two aspects of exposure to *L. tropica* and resulting infection with leishmania: the occurrence of either cutaneous or visceral leishmaniasis; and the possibility that some component of unexplained illness may result from leishmania infection.

One investigator has estimated that 5 to 6 percent of Gulf War veterans are infected with leishmania, which can lead to chronic illness (Magill, 1994). Leishmania have incubation periods from months to years. The organism may persist in the host after treatment that appears to be effective; thus relapse is not uncommon. Illness results from a cellular immune response that produces cytokine mediated symptoms that are compatible with some of the symptoms reported as part of the GWS; these also have been produced by giving interferon gamma to healthy persons. Thus, some observers have concluded that GWS could result from visceral leishmaniasis among soldiers who participated in Operation Desert Storm. Because the presentation of illness associated with *L. tropica* infection does not fit the classical presentation of visceral leishmaniasis, it is referred to as viscerotropic leishmaniasis. Two issues raised by the eight known, documented cases of viscerotropic leishmaniasis in returning Desert Storm troops are the late presentation due to prolonged incubation and the activation of latent infection in immunosupressed persons. Latent leishmania can be a problem in persons with HIV, after organ transplantation, and during administration of high doses of corticosteroids. If *L. tropica* can survive in a latent state, it will need to be included in differential diagnoses of otherwise unexplained illnesses in returning veterans from Operation Desert Storm (Cotton, 1992; Kreutzer et al., 1993; Lesho, 1991; Magill et al., 1993; MMWR, 1992; Norton et al., 1992; Ohl et al., 1993; Rashti et al., 1992).

HEALTH-OUTCOME-BASED ACTIVITIES-NEW OR JUST BEGINNING

Issues of Reproductive Health

Illness and toxic agents can affect reproductive health in many ways (Mattison, 1994). One outcome of great concern is birth defects. Two types of approaches could be used to determine whether birth defects are related to parental service in the Persian Gulf. The first is to identify and study all putative exposures likely to produce transmissible genetic defects or adverse health effects in a fetus or newborn. Fathers' exposures could be studied in relation to the genetic defects (sperm-mediated); and mothers' exposures could be related to either genetic or developmental defects (mediated by the ovum or through *in utero* exposures). The second is to compare all children with some adverse health outcome with a suitable set of controls to establish the location and status of each parent before, at the time of, and after conception, whether or not the defect was genetic or consistent with known toxicity of the potential exposure.

Reproductive health outcomes linked to Persian Gulf War service have been noted prominently in the news media, but have received only limited scientific attention. To date, there are two evaluations that are complete or nearly complete: The Mississippi Cluster Study and a review of Army data by the Army Surgeon General's Office (PGVCB, 1994).

The Mississippi cluster study involved evaluating 54 birth outcomes of the Army Reserve Unit of Waynesboro, Mississippi. The final report should be available by December 1994. The preliminary conclusions of the report are that the birth defect rates were not elevated compared with those in the Metropolitan Atlanta Congenital Defects Program (Mississippi State Department of Health, 1994).

In the Army Surgeon General's evaluation of major and minor birth defects of active duty personnel at all Army hospitals from 1985 to 1993 (n = 346,322), rates of major and minor defects ranged from 5.8 percent to 9.6 percent with 8 percent to 17 percent expected from comparison with the Metropolitan Atlanta Congenital Defects Program. Rates for 1992 and 1993 (following the Gulf War) were similar. Only births in Army hospitals to active duty women or spouses of active duty service members were included. These data reflect birth defects recognized at the time of discharge after birth (after 2 to 3 days of age). Thus, the data would underascertain minor malformations and conditions detected later in infancy.

Neither of these two studies has revealed an incidence of birth defects that differs from expected rates. General Accounting Office (GAO) review (GAO, 1994) of the Mississippi cluster study has questioned whether the Atlanta birth defects database is an appropriate comparison group, and whether rates of birth defects would be reduced if the Mississippi veterans were selectively healthier than the Atlanta database parents. They also recommended that the predeployment incidence of birth defects be assessed and used as a comparison.

Likewise, reviewers of the DoD study have noted that births to active duty military personnel occur outside DoD hospitals, and that infertility and miscarriages constitute important outcomes of reproductive toxicant exposures that are not included in the DoD database.

A new initiative, the DoD Reproductive Health Study, contains data from hospital records of active duty personnel and spouses for whom the discharge diagnoses include fetal death, premature birth, serious birth defect, or neonatal death (CDR Gregory Gray, 1994, personal communication). Records from the DoD hospitalizations of 350,000 Persian Gulf veterans and 700,000 personnel not deployed in that era will be examined. A recent update (September 7, 1994) from the project director indicates that a survey will be conducted of 20,000 couples to assess miscarriage and infertility frequency. This reproductive health study was not yet begun at the writing of this report (September 1994).

Surveillance of reproductive health is included in the DoD and VA clinical examinations. Information obtained by the VA Health Registry examination includes data about birth defects among children conceived before and after Gulf War deployment. Miscarriage and infertility data were added after the first 20,000 surveys were completed; it is uncertain whether the VA will go back to obtain infertility and miscarriage data from the first 20,000 participants. Information obtained by the DoD includes data similar to that in the VA Health Registry exam. Despite these efforts, the ability to link exposures to reproductive health outcomes will be limited for each of these databases. At this time, high-quality population-based data on reproductive health have not been generated.

VA Mortality Study Plans

The VA has indicated plans to retrospectively compare the causes of mortality of all Persian Gulf War veterans to that of Persian Gulf War-era veterans who did not serve in the Persian Gulf theater. The study population of approximately 690,000 will be defined by service in the Persian Gulf theater of operations at any time between August 1990 and April 1991. The Persian Gulf-era veterans will be a sample of military personnel who served at any time between September 1990 and May 1991, but did not serve in the Persian Gulf theater. The controls will be frequency-matched to the Persian Gulf veterans by branch of service and unit status.

Mortality will be ascertained using the VA Beneficiary Identification and Records Locator Subsystem (BIRLS), Social Security Administration records, and the National Death Index (NDI). The follow-up period will begin for Persian Gulf veterans on the day they left the Persian Gulf area alive, or May 1, 1991, whichever is earlier. Controls will be followed beginning May 1, 1991. Follow-up for mortality ascertainment will end either on the date of death, or September 31, 1993, whichever came first.

This study will be useful in determining whether there are any unusual acute mortality causes in veterans of the Persian Gulf War, as compared with veterans of the same era who did not serve in the Persian Gulf; however, insufficient time has passed to observe any excess mortality from chronic diseases.

VA Health Survey Study Plans

The VA has indicated plans to conduct a health survey to estimate the prevalence of various symptoms and other health outcomes among Persian Gulf veterans and Persian Gulf-era veterans and their spouses and children in relation to certain environmental exposures. The study will include a population-based sample of 15,000 Persian Gulf veterans and an equal number of Persian Gulf-era veterans. This will be a mail survey, supplemented by telephone interviews and physical examination (Health Registry Exam) of a sample of veterans. The study is proposed to be validated through military and VA records.

We hope that the investigators will employ sophisticated statistical sampling techniques to ensure that the study and control populations are properly selected, and that procedures are used to ensure the representativeness and precision of the estimates to be obtained. There are several concerns about this proposed study. Mailed questionnaires are known to have very poor response rates; therefore, the investigators should try to obtain an adequate response rate that is nondifferential in the two groups. Otherwise, there is a high probability that such a study will produce neither reliable estimates of symptoms and other health outcomes, nor estimates that represent the actual experience of either group of veterans. The potential for response bias is great, with PG veterans having problems being more likely to respond than those who do not. Additionally, a tally of symptoms and illnesses will get no closer to understanding whether any of these problems occurred *because of* some experience or exposure related to PG service.

Iowa Study

At the initiation of Senator Tom Harkin of Iowa, the Centers for Disease Control and Prevention (CDC) will conduct a study to assess the prevalence of self-reported adverse health outcomes among Iowa residents deployed to the Persian Gulf during ODS and deployed elsewhere. Of the 20,000 Iowa residents who served in the Gulf War, 3,500 were reservists or National Guard members and 16,800 were on active duty. Current plans call for the study sample to include approximately 2,000 Persian Gulf veterans and PG-era veterans, both men and women, and will include active duty, reserve, and national guard personnel who listed Iowa as their home of residence. The research group plans to use telephone survey methods to assess factors that can be classified as preservice (health status, psychosocial functioning, trauma exposure), service (perceived stress, combat experiences, actual duties, perceived exposures, prior military experience) and post-service (health status, psychosocial functioning, PTSD, depression, chronic fatigue). A more detailed study proposal was not available at this writing (September 1994).

What specific gaps in knowledge will be addressed by this study is unclear, as is whether there is any scientific basis for a study restricted to the veterans of Iowa or any other single state. Whatever other merits, this study seems unlikely to produce useful new medical or scientific information about the health effects of service in the PG. This is because of the relatively small number of veterans included, limited geographical distribution, possible biases in geographic dispersion or in the initial characteristics of veterans from Iowa, difficulty in obtaining information on deceased veterans identified for the study population, and lack of organized expert attention to study design. A single state is unlikely to represent the national experience. There is no reason to believe that Iowa veterans have more problems than others or merit more attention. State-by-state reviews are neither productive nor informative.

DoD/VA Studies of Morbidity among Gulf War Veterans

Researchers at the Naval Health Research Center, San Diego, California have developed a protocol with three primary components: 1) a survey of symptoms among 1,500 Seabee veterans who participated in the PGW and 750 who did not participate; 2) a comparison of hospitalizations among 350,000 PG veterans (Navy, Marine, and Army), with those of 700,000 persons not deployed; and 3) a review of adverse pregnancy outcomes among both PG veterans and persons not in the war, as reported at discharge from Army hospitals (Gray, 1994).

This is a well-funded enterprise of nearly three million dollars over a five-year project period. The investigators have described their general methods, but the details of the protocols are still being revised. As of this writing, the IOM committee has not received or reviewed a final protocol for these studies.

The studies address important questions and proceed logically. There will be an analysis of self-reported symptoms, hospitalizations, and pregnancies, which will make good use of available data. Incomplete follow-up is a threat to data quality, especially when it is related to an outcome of interest. Thus, there should be a tracking system to follow participants who leave military service.

Key concerns are the baseline comparability of persons who did and did not serve in the PGW. The investigators propose to look at this, and careful and detailed assessment is central to the enterprise. Any notable discrepancies will need to be addressed by stratification and adjustment, and all of these will need a sensitivity analysis. This concern is no different from that in all observational studies, but data on some relevant variables might not be available to the researchers, and some variables might not even be known to be important.

Data on an individual's exposures related to PGW service are an important aspect of the study, and it remains to be seen how well exposures can be estimated from available data. In fact, the major strength of these studies may lie in uncovering a dose-response (exposure-response) relationship among PG veterans in relation to specific exposures, rather than in comparing those who did serve against those who did not. Also, persons who did not go to the Persian Gulf may not be a valid control group, even after adjustment for a wide variety of preservice imbalances.

The studies are complex scientifically and organizationally. Follow-up of selected samples can be very informative, provided the follow-up is accurate, detailed, and sufficiently complete. It is not clear that the project has the infrastructure or staff to ensure success. Additionally, attention needs to be given to the issue of career military service versus reserve status, particularly because the current indications concerning GWS focus primarily among the reservists who are not included in this set of studies. The proposed five-year duration of this study seems too short to detect cancers, though it may be longer than is necessary for observing more acute effects. In all of the studies, primary attention should be paid to collecting reliable data, and documenting problems with the data sets, which should be communicated to other researchers in a timely manner. Some details of the individually proposed studies follow:

Seabees Study

This study will assess health conditions, environmental exposures, and potential confounders among 2,250 active Seabees (two battalions of a total of 1,500 PG veterans and one battalion of 750 who were not deployed to the

Gulf). Data are to come primarily from an interview that is designed to identify clinical, occupational, geographical, temporal, and demographic risk factors. Data from computerized hospital records, unit diaries, and PG veterans registries will be available. Limited physical examination will be done. Whole blood and serum samples will be stored for future analysis; urine samples will be collected and stored; and a lung function test will be done.

Missing information is likely to cause an assessment problem in this portion of the study. If only active duty Seabees are included in the study, bias is likely. If not, there must be prompt and detailed decisions about how discharged persons are to be found. An added concern is whether the Seabees will provide accurate information. With the current military reduction in forces, there may be a tendency to under-report problems to protect their jobs. This should not, however, affect the assessment of physical signs or laboratory findings unless persons with problems have a low participation rate as well as biased reporting of symptoms.

Hospitalization Study

A computerized hospitalization discharge database will be used to study 350,000 PGW personnel who are still in active service. With respect to hospitalizations after July 1991. these persons will be compared with a randomly selected cohort of 700,000 soldiers not deployed to the Persian Gulf The investigators will assess pre-PGW health status, and will try to track persons who leave the military, and capture information on their hospitalizations.

Again, missing information is likely to cause an assessment problem in this portion of the study. Hospitalizations of only persons still on active duty are likely to be a biased identification of the sick population. Also there is the concern that methods have not been determined to track persons discharged from the service. The possible differential tendency of PGW veterans and those not in the war to seek care outside the military system is a further threat to the study. Some of these concerns are addressed by the addition of the California nonfederal hospitalization component that will obtain information from nonmilitary hospitals.

The hospital database should be quite accurate and complete regarding the fact of hospitalization, but data on specific diagnoses, symptoms, and signs may be much less accurate and complete. There is a good data system for evaluating the hospitalization of active duty service personnel; however, these data systems do not track non-DoD hospitalizations and outpatient visits.

Pregnancy Outcome Study

The women studied for pregnancy outcomes (fetal death, premature birth, serious birth defects, and neonatal deaths) will be a subset of the hospitalization study. This study has been mentioned above in the section entitled "Reproductive Health."

There are likely to be problems in the assessment of pregnancy outcomes, particularly specific birth defects, based on routinely available hospital records. Similarly, gestational age estimates will be subject to error. Nevertheless, given the scarcity of informative data on reproductive health outcomes among PG veterans, either completed or in progress, analyses of available data are justified.

ASSESSMENTS OF EXPOSURE

Environmental

Only limited information is available to study possible links between environmental exposures and the unusual medical conditions that have been reported to be associated with service in the Persian Gulf War. While environmental exposures may have been important, the data needed for sound epidemiological study are very limited. Of data available, the most reliable findings seem to refer to oil well fires and lead. However, the information is skimpy for several reasons. First, there was minimal systematic sampling and measuring of possible environmental hazards; even expert descriptions of environments rarely are available. Also, the wide range of health outcomes that some persons have attributed to service in the Persian Gulf have yet to be grouped into useful and biologically plausible categories. Therefore, it is premature to narrow the consideration of exposures to specific agents or different types of environments. In addition, the vast majority of the health investigations that the committee reviewed were neither designed around one or several precise hypotheses nor based on well-characterized "populations at risk." Therefore, the consideration of types of exposures potentially important with respect to the reported problems can be presented only in a general way.

The environment that veterans encountered in the Persian Gulf is usefully considered in two categories: general and occupational. General environmental exposures of interest include temperature and humidity, sand and dirt, sanitary conditions, fauna, oil well spills and fires, pesticides, petroleum products (especially jet fuel and diesel fuel containing lead additives), mycotoxins, and decontamination solution. Exposures to consider under occupational environment are related mainly to general maintenance operations and include battery repair, cleaning/degreasing, electronic/radio repair, generator repair, grinding/sanding, sand blasting, lathing/milling, painting (especially with isocyanate-based paints), refrigeration servicing, vehicle repair, weapons repair, and welding and cutting.

General Environment

An adequate description of the general environmental conditions is still being developed. The following is a summary of the information available at the time of writing (September 1994).

Temperature and Humidity.

Mean daily low and high temperatures were 80°F and 108°F in July, and 45°F and 65°F in the winter. Except in coastal regions, the relative humidity was less than 40 percent during the summer, but over 60 percent during the rainy season (December through March). Solar heat was intense in the summer. Rain was minimal (3 to 8 inches) but sometimes caused the flooding of tents (DSB, 1994).

Sand and Dirt.

Most troops were located in desert settings where sand was ubiquitous. The sand often was powdery, and persons with respiratory conditions sometimes reported respiratory symptoms. Whether these symptoms were properly attributed to sand rather than to the type of living structure (tent versus air-conditioned building), or other problem has not been determined (DSB, 1994).

Sanitary Conditions.

Sanitary conditions in the Gulf theater need a systematic review that is not yet possible from available records. However, the following has been reported as a summary of the sanitary conditions.

> Staging areas near ports of entry were characterized by crowded tent living with strains on latrine facilities, showers, and feeding. The prototype four-scat latrines were mass produced by contract in country. Latrines were designed for suction removal of waste by contractors or bum-out. Early designs permitted ingress of flies. In the desert environment, daily burning out of waste cans employed mainly diesel fuel. Smoke from such fires was common, though rapidly dispersed by prevailing winds. Solid waste disposal was handled by contract in the staging areas and by burning in pits in the desert. Locations for burn pits and latrines were usually chosen carefully to minimize nuisance from smoke, smells, and flies. When shower/bath units were not available, many field expedients were improvised. Likewise for laundry. As shower setups became available or were improvised, an unforeseen problem was heating the water once the cooler weather set in. Time in

tervals between showers and uniform laundering were sometimes lengthy (O'Donnell, 1994).

Food and Water.

The final report of the United States Army Environmental Hygiene Agency (USAEHA) does not contain a discussion of the possibility that troops were exposed to contaminated water or food. This is because local drinking water was not used. The troops and civilians were provided with sealed containers of drinking water; food was provided in the form of meals ready-to-eat (MREs) sealed in plastic, or provided at the mess hall. Personnel generally did not eat food produced from the local areas. This helped prevent diarrheal illness. In all previous military engagements, diarrheal disease was a major problem; therefore, incidence was surprisingly lower in PGW. In addition, "there was no reason to believe that the local food was contaminated with oil fire residue" (USAEHA, 1994a).

Fauna.

Exposures to fauna also need a systemic review that is not possible at this time. The following has been reported as a summary of certain exposures.

> Filth flies were a universal problem in the warm months. Latrines and food sources were attractants. The use of screening, self-closing doors, fly traps, fly bait, and pesticides were moderately successful suppressants. Various types of scorpions and snakes such as the horned viper were common in the desert, and envenomation of personnel occurred occasionally. Although biting spiders were present, they were not a problem. Mosquitoes were a factor only in the Euphrates Valley. Sandflies were present, as evidenced by the cases of leishmaniasis, but were difficult to find even when searched for. Sheep and camels were commonly observed in the desert. Dead sheep were often reported, but veterinary inquiries disclosed no signs of unexpected causes of death. Unit pets or mascots were officially banned but some small units adopted stray dogs and obtained veterinary care through Saudi sources (O'Donnell, 1994).

The report that no signs of unexpected causes of death among sheep or camels were noted is not consistent with a report the committee received in the public meeting, where one veteran described his investigation of an episode of widespread unexplained sheep deaths (IOM public meeting, March 1, 1994).

Pesticides.

DoD apparently has or could produce a listing of all pesticides shipped to the Persian Gulf, but the committee knows of no central record of their distribution and use. The following are the pesticides reported as likely to have been used at some time in some locations: allethrin/resmethrin, azamethiphos, bendiocarb, chlorphyrifos, diazinon, malathion, d-phenothrin, permethrin, and pyrethrin. There are no reports of the use of herbicides and no reports of acute pesticide poisonings. Summary information indicates that pesticides were generally applied either using one-or two-gallon sprayers or directly by hand. There was also an indication that marines did some "ultra low volume fogging" (PGVCB, 1994). The virtual absence of reports of sandfly fever suggests that vector control was in general good (Richards et al., 1991; Richards et al., 1993).

Petroleum Products.

Many different fuels were used in the Persian Gulf to power vehicles and for heaters, cooking stoves, and portable generators. The exhaust produced in the course of using these fuels (particularly the use of diesel heaters in living quarters) could have caused a variety of exposures to combustion products including lead. Even though there are several accounts of exposure to these sources, the committee has not received information either to directly evaluate the likelihood that such sources resulted in important exposure to the troops or to determine levels of exposures (either substance-specific or through measurements of surrogates or indicators for the exhaust gases). It appears that approval of the use of diesel fuel for firing stoves was based on work undertaken at the Natick Research and Development Center before the Gulf War (Riley, 1992).

Decontamination Solution.

The committee found only one reference to the decontamination solution for the treatment of equipment exposed to chemical warfare agents, which stated the following:

> Decontamination Solution 2 (DS-2) is a liquid mixture to decontaminate equipment that has been exposed to chemical warfare agents. The constituents are propylene glycol monomethyl ether or ethylene glycol, sodium hydroxide, and diethylenetriamine. DS-2 does not seem to have produced widespread problems in the Persian Gulf region and chronic effects after a single exposure are still conjectural (PGVCB, 1994).

Oil Well Spills and Fires

Several efforts have been made to determine whether the oil well spills and fires created by the retreating Iraqi forces caused any health effects among U.S. troops. These effects have been summarized by USAEHA (USAEHA, 1992; USAEHA, 1994a). They include Kuwait and Saudi environmental assessments; reports from EPA (EPA, 1991), France, and Great Britain that were beginning or completed in March and April of 1991; reports from Japan and Harvard University beginning or completed in April; reports from the National Institute of Standards and Technology, the National Center for Atmospheric Research, Norway, and Germany beginning or completed in May; reports beginning or completed in June from the National Oceanographic and Atmospheric Administration (NOAA)/Air Resources Lab; reports beginning or completed in July from EPA/National Aeronautics and Space Administration (NASA) and Lawrence Livermore Labs; and reports from Germany in October. The Defense Nuclear Agency carried out some ground-based measurements during an unknown period. The interim USAEHA report provides very limited information about these studies and none about the deoxyribonucleic acid (DNA) study. The final USAEHA report suggests that further examination of these reports, along with the published literature on the fires, will be done in conjunction with the Geographical Information System (GIS) project, which is still in process.

The major effort at environmental assessment was undertaken by USAEHA to evaluate troop exposures to the oil well fires and oil spills. While exposures began when the first oil well fires were ignited in February 1991 by the Iraq armed forces during their retreat and lasted until November 1, 1991, USAEHA's air sampling effort could not be successfully launched until the beginning of May. Therefore, the more stagnant air conditions of the winter months were missed. Those who undertook the sampling efforts did so with this knowledge and intended to address the problem as well as possible by the use of meteorological modeling. A GIS is being developed to integrate information on airborne and soil-based exposures, on meteorological conditions throughout the study interval, and on individual troop movements during Operation Desert Storm. Results from a pilot project in developing the GIS indicate that the approach should prove useful (USAEHA, 1994a). Once this model is available, individual exposure estimates can be made for troops throughout the region, though further work will still be needed to validate the model and estimate its precision.

At the maximum there were ten fixed air-sampling stations, but two of them operated for less than two weeks and two more operated for two months. Only three were in operation through the end of December.

These fixed sites were located where troops were concentrated, and soil was sampled from the same areas. The results are to be used with NOAA-assisted modeling to estimate reasonable maximum individual exposures (RMEs) to the chemical substances sampled according to records of troop movements using the GIS. These included air and soil pathway analysis and industrial hygiene sampling. Air and soil quality was estimated not to have deteriorated during the sampling interval, and a reference to earlier sampling suggests that quality at some sites was even higher than before the war. Soil metals did not increase during sampling except for metals unrelated to Kuwaiti crude oil.

The air pollutants expected were classified into four categories: reactants (crude oil components not combusted); combustion products (such as carbon dioxide and water); incomplete combustion products (for example, carbon monoxide), and products of secondary reactions (from photolysis). The substances included short-chain and low-and medium-molecular weight aliphatics such as butane and heptane (both straight and branch chain in the range C_2 to C_{40}); single and polycyclic aromatic hydrocarbons (PAHs); heterocyclic compounds including benzene, naphthalene, and xylene; and substituted compounds such as methylated and halogenated compounds. Samples were assayed for suspended particulates, both total and particulate matter less than 10 microns, a series of volatile organics, PAHs, and metals. A subsample was examined for sulfur dioxide, nitrogen dioxide, coal-tar pitch volatiles, and acid aerosols. These agents were chosen as likely to provide a reasonable estimate of the impact of the oil well fires and spills. The sampling results were designed for use in estimates of cancer risk and subchronic, noncancer risk.

As yet, none of the agents sampled or detected are obvious sources of problems that would cause persistent symptoms for months or years after return from the Persian Gulf. The modeling may, however, offer some improved understanding of the differences in the general environment of troops located in different parts of the war zone.

The most striking outcome of the USAEHA sampling and the report of the EPA sampling is that there was very little documented deterioration of general air quality during the period of the burning oil wells and oil spills. The only substantial increase noted was in particulates. The concentration of particulates, while high, was considered "normal" for this area of the Middle East. Exposures to organic compounds were similar to levels observed in Houston and Philadelphia, cities with major petrochemical industries. There were relatively high concentrations of naturally occurring metals, apparently resulting from wind-blown surface soils. The levels of air pollution were high enough to raise concerns about ingestion and dermal absorption, and these routes of exposure have been considered (USAEHA, 1994a). However, no measurements were taken, so that the possible effects of exposure through these additional routes can be estimated only by mathematical models.

When individual exposures can be estimated, the effects of different levels of exposures to pollution from the oil fires can be estimated by using troop location during the largest part of the time in the Persian Gulf region. For example, the prevailing winds (from northwest in Kuwait and from north-northwest in Saudi Arabia) should have caused substantial differences in potential exposure of troops, because some troops were both close and downwind; others were either distant or to the side of the prevailing windflow.

Further work by USAEHA is expected to provide a model of the exposure distributions and incorporate information from earlier, more limited sampling that might improve the estimates of exposures to troop encampments. The work by USAEHA also will examine the frequency and duration of exposures. When this information is available, the time course of symptoms in different troops could usefully be studied.

In summary, these assessments of exposures to products of the torched and destroyed oil wells will apparently include information on relatively low-level exposures to a variety of petroleum-related chemical substances. It will then be possible—and important—to consider more specific questions about symptoms and health outcomes, including any effects of troop location and troop movement, and the time-courses of each of these. Because accurate information on exposure of individual persons is not available, epidemiological assessment of differences in illness or symptoms reported by different troops in various locations holds the greatest promise for indicating health problems related to chemical exposures.

Biologic Surveillance

"Small groups" from the 11th Armored Cavalry Regiment were surveyed in June, August, and October of 1991 before, during, and after 90-day deployment from Germany to Kuwait (USAEHA, 1994b). Tests included questionnaires on symptoms, moods, exposures, and work; a pulmonary function test; blood samples for metals, volatile compounds, and sister chromatid exchanges (SCEs); and urinary measures for metals and benzo-a-pyrene (BaP). Approximately 2,800 of 4,700 troops volunteered to complete a questionnaire in predeployment, 350 during service in the Persian Gulf, and 1,700 post-deployment. There is no evidence of a change in pulmonary function, although the predeployment values did not meet technical standards for usability. Serum and urine tests for metals were carried out in 150 to 175 persons in the three periods; for volatile organic chemicals (VOCs) in 28 to 32 persons; for SCEs in 3,661 and for PAH-DNA in 34 to 42. Some increase in symptoms was reported in the Persian Gulf. Metal analysis was remarkable only for a slight and nonsignificant increase in the average level of blood lead. Elevations were noted in a minority of the troops, suggesting that a local rather than a general explanation should be sought. No ready explanation for this increase has been provided, though lead exposures from the use of diesel fuels for tent heating were apparently not considered. Nickel (Ni) and vanadium (V) (present in Kuwaiti crude oil) were not elevated. VOCs have a very short half-life in the body, and therefore their measurements relate to very recent exposure. The VOCs were, in general, lower during the time in the Persian Gulf than before or after, with the exception of a small, unexplained elevation in perchlorethylene. Since perchlorethylene is a chlorinated hydrocarbon it was thought that blood level increases were unlikely to be caused by exposure to oil well fires. Acetone levels seemed to have been slightly elevated, but still need to be examined for normalcy. SCE levels were elevated during time in the Persian Gulf; PAH-DNA adducts were lower during service there than either pre-or post-deployment. Even though the elevated SCE levels were evidence of some genetic stress, no source of such stress has been identified. The reduced levels of PAH-DNA were attributed to unusually low exposures during service in the Persian Gulf Analysis of urinary tetrols and overall data analysis is continuing.

Autopsy Studies

Some battlefield casualties were further examined at autopsy for possible connections between exposures and mortality or morbidity. The Armed Forces Institute of Pathology examined 85 corpses of troops who died in the Gulf War theater. Some were autopsied, some had only a study of body fluids, and some had both studies. These included deaths both before and after smoke exposure.

Blood was examined for contaminants, mostly heavy metals: V, Ni, chromium (Cr), lead (Pb), copper (Cu), and zinc (Zn). Autopsy findings did not suggest acute pulmonary, liver, or renal failure. Except for expected pathology nothing unusual was seen. Because the smoke from the oil fires contained V and Ni, a finding of excess V or Ni would suggest exposure. No such excess was found. However, in seven cases, a high blood Pb level was seen:

Case	Pb μg/dl
910120	63.2*
910216	99.2*
910217	110.5*
910223	29.7
910358	148.3*
910397	71.3*
910499	32.2

These tests (*) were thought to be contaminated because of the high value. The author indicated that the normal range was 7 to 19, with an average of 12.5 (AFIP, 1993). Although isotope studies of the samples might help, it is impossible to determine whether there was contamination. However, these reported high measurements are compatible with acute lead poisoning, such as might occur from burning leaded diesel fuel in heaters in unvented sleeping tents. These high values might indicate substantial exposures in the staging area. Also, the elevated blood lead levels might indicate higher exposures to a variety of petroleum combustion and evaporation contaminates. If surviving troops suffered from acute lead poisoning, blood lead levels today would not be abnormal, but X-ray florescence might show that blood and bone levels are still increased. Troops might still be asked about transient gastrointestinal pain immediately after exposure. Despite the purported negative findings, the paucity of the above data, and its non-scientific format would still not permit any conclusions about toxicity.

Occupational Environment

Little summary information has been identified that characterizes the range of occupational exposures that may have occurred in the Persian Gulf beyond those that might be associated with the occupation of "soldier." It appears that the majority of possible occupational exposures would be related mainly to repair and maintenance activities to keep equipment in functional order. No information is currently available on the numbers of troops who were assigned regularly or intermittently to the different components of support work in the Persian Gulf.

Because the operating conditions were far from ideal, and the environments generally were not sufficiently fixed for adherence to recommended occupational hygiene controls, some of these exposures could have been substantial. Trained industrial hygienists in the Gulf reported that exposures in fixed work environments generally could have been kept within current standards there, but that operations in the field may not have allowed sufficiently stringent controls (Riley, 1992). This was particularly the case for painting operations that called for laminar flow hoods. Personal protective equipment was a key feature of adequate exposure control in painting operations. The industrial hygiene staff used the American Conference of Governmental Industrial Hygienists' (ACGIH) Threshold Limit Values (TLVs) as their primary guide. Commentary indicates that these limits were considered sufficient to protect against any health effects (USAEHA, 1992). However, Rappaport (1993) has shown that many of these limits are based on feasibility rather than on protecting against all health effects.

The following listing includes most of the potential chemical hazards associated with common maintenance or repair operations. With the exception of vehicle painting, information on actual exposure evaluations for these work settings is not available. Therefore, the operations that are likely to have occurred are characterized primarily by noting the potential chemical exposure risks.

- Battery Repair: Corrosive liquids, particularly sulfuric acid, lead.
- Cleaning/Degreasing: Degreasing solvents generally including a range of chlorinated hydrocarbons such as trichloroethylene.
- Electronic/Radio Repair: Soldering fumes and cleaning solvents.
- Generator Repair: Carbon monoxide.
- Grinding/Sanding: Abrasive particulate.
- Sand blasting: Abrasive (possibly crystalline silica) particulates in the respirable range.
- Lathing/Milling: Metal working fluids.
- Vehicle Painting: Paint solvent vapors and mists. During primary and repair painting operations there was a potential for overexposure to isocyanate paints, which can cause primary sensitization and asthma as well as exacerbation of existing asthma. The chemical agent resistant coating (CARC) paint system was directly used by an estimated 1,000 troops (PGVCB, 1994). The number of vehicles painted each day varied between 10 and 100 at the major work site in Al Jabayl. At least one episode of overexposure was reported (December, 1990) (Riley, 1992).
- Refrigeration servicing: Lead fumes and exposure to refrigerant such as fluorocarbons.
- Vehicle Repair: Asbestos from brake repair, carbon monoxide, organic solvents.
- Weapons Repair: Lead particulate.
- Welding/Cutting: Chromates, ozone, nitrogen dioxides, heated metal fumes.

USAEHA industrial hygiene sampling showed increases in personal or general air monitoring results of outdoor occupational environment from selected locations, but these increased levels still did not exceed recommended standards.

Threat of Chemical and Biological Warfare Agents

Direct and indirect statements to this committee by several Gulf War veterans and groups speaking on their behalf have ranged from worried concern to firm statements that troops were exposed to unspecified war agents, chemical, biological, or both. The strong suspicions seem to be that exposures were to nerve agents stockpiled by the Iraqis for use against Iran and the Kurdish population. Such stockpiling and use would have preceded Operation Desert Storm. Some claims have also been made that U.S. CDC Type-Cultures (anthrax and botulism) supplied by the United States to Iraq in the 1980's for research and vaccine production could have been fashioned into weapons and used, overtly or covertly, against U.S. forces. Testimony before several Congressional committees has carried into the press strong assertions that members of Congress or their staffs actually have concluded that self-reported signs and symptoms said to be associated with soviet-designed surface-to-surface missiles (SCUD) attacks and concomitant chemical and biological warfare (CBW) alarms were sufficiently convincing to make a *prime facie* case for CBW use. These assertions have been amply reported elsewhere in the public domain and will not be repeated here.

The committee could find absolutely no reliable intelligence, and no medical or biological justification for any of these purported claims. Furthermore, analysis of the attacks indicated that the alarms were false positives generated by dust particulates. When analysis of the alarms was followed by more sophisticated tests, the results were confirmed to be negative. This information speaks convincingly against the claims of CBW. Official analyses by the Central Intelligence Agency (CIA) Directorate of Intelligence, the CIA Non-Proliferation Center, the Defense Intelligence Agency, and a high-level all-source DoD committee, the Task Force of the Defense Science Board have concluded, independently and based on all-source/codeword access, that no use by intention or by accident occurred, and that bombing of storage areas both in theater and to the rear also did not cause CBW exposure. These reports are also in the public domain and will not be further referenced here.

One member of the IOM committee obtained classified briefings on known Iraqi capabilities, believed intentions, and prior use of weapons of mass destruction. The committee as a whole obtained briefings on theater operations and CBW suspicions. This material was obtained and reviewed prior to and after disclosure and declassification of most of the same material and the committee found no inconsistencies. This material is now in the public domain and will not be further referenced here.

The committee is not aware of any other actual data, complete or incomplete, that are inconsistent with the above conclusions and is not aware of any reports or studies, classified or unclassified that are inconsistent with the above. Therefore, the committee believes that the illnesses that have been reported are not the result of chemical, biological, or toxin warfare, or accidental exposures to stored weapons or research material. The committee believes further that, in light of this negative evidence from highly placed sources, claims of exposure to chemical or biological warfare agents should not be made or given credence in the absence of reliable data to the contrary.

Vaccines and Prophylactic Treatment

Anthrax and Botulinum Toxoid

The threat of CBW was quite real, as mentioned above, when troops were deployed. Threats of chemical and biological warfare were anticipated. DoD vaccinated some troops against anthrax and botulism, which were considered the biological warfare agents most likely to be encountered. These vaccines were not administered together. Individuals receiving vaccines signed their consent to a list. Prophylactic treatment against possible chemical warfare agents was provided in the form of self-administered pills.

Respiratory-acquired anthrax is a fatal disease unless the diagnosis is made and appropriate antibiotic treatment is begun within hours of exposure. Botulism is a fatal disease caused by potent neurotoxins released by *Clostridium botulinum* that must be promptly neutralized by antitoxin therapy. There was concern that the Iraqi forces could use one or both of these agents against U.S. forces during ODS. Vaccines against them were made available to selected groups. Several factors have created questions about these vaccines: they were unique in the military immunization program; the botulism toxoid was distributed to the Army as an investigational new drug (IND) by the Food and Drug Administration (FDA) and was to be given on a voluntary basis with informed consent; the anthrax program was involuntary; many persons believed that these vaccines were not properly tested; the program was classified as secret; and each vaccine was intended to prevent serious disease induced by these potential biological weapons. These concerns have raised further questions about a possible role of these vaccines in the long-term health effects reported by some recipients.

Anthrax vaccine contains the known protective antigen of a killed avirulent strain of *Bacillus anthracis*. In order to enhance its immunogenicity, it is absorbed onto an adjuvant, aluminum hydroxide. The vaccine has been produced by the Michigan State Department of Public Health and licensed since 1972. The primary nonmilitary use has been for persons with occupational risks—those workers who process wool, goat hair, animal hides, and bone and bone products. It has also been administered to laboratory workers. Over 7,900 doses have been given in the past 22 years to employees at the U.S. Army Medical Research Institute of Infectious Diseases (USAMRIID).

The recommended dosage schedule of anthrax vaccine is 6 injections over an 18-month period. Few service members in ODS received more than the first 2 doses, given 2 weeks apart. The program was discontinued when the war was over. It is estimated that about 150,000 service members received at least one dose. The known side-effects of the vaccine include tenderness, erythema, and swelling at the injection site. These have been reported in about

6 percent of recipients. Less that 1 percent have more severe local reactions, which may limit the use of the arm for 1 to 2 days. Systemic reactions rarely have been reported, and no chronic sequelae have been noted. The reaction rates among those receiving the vaccine in ODS were unmeasured. One person was hospitalized because of an infection at the injection site.

Botulinum toxoid vaccine consists of five of the most common types of toxins (A, B, C, D, E) that have been toxoided by use of formalin. It is also manufactured by the Michigan State Department of Public Health. Alum is used as an adjuvant. Botulinum toxoid vaccine has status as an IND with the FDA, as mentioned, and has been used as an investigational vaccine for over 20 years. More than 3,600 doses have been administered at USAMRIID. This experience has permitted an estimate of the reaction rate. There have been more mild local reactions (up to 10 percent) than noted with anthrax vaccine, and about 3 percent experienced mild systemic reactions, such as headache, myalgia, fever, and malaise for 48 to 72 hours. No chronic sequelae have been reported.

The vaccine is to be given in 3 injections: an initial dose, followed by other injections at 2 and 12 weeks, with a booster at 1 year. About 8,000 service members received at least 1 dose. The recipients were primarily members of the U.S. Marine Corps, First Marine Division, and the U.S. Army VII Corps. None of those troops received the anthrax vaccine. All members of these units were to have had the opportunity to volunteer and to give informed consent before receiving the vaccine. No reaction data were collected. A retrospective postcard survey was conducted at Camp Pendleton for the Marines who received the vaccine. Of the 123 cards mailed, 121 responded. Of respondents, 96 percent had received 2 doses; 12 percent reported mild local reactions; 14 percent reported pain that limited use of the arm temporarily; and 2.5 percent reported systemic symptoms that did not limit activity. There was no evidence of long-term effects.

The military has had long experience with vaccine administration. There are 7 vaccines administered during basic training to Army recruits. All active duty Army personnel receive one additional vaccine, as well as boosters to two of the basic training immunizations. Seven other vaccines, excluding anthrax and botulinum toxoids, are given for deployment to high-risk areas, to alert forces, as required by host country, or as directed by the surgeon general. Each of these 15 vaccines can produce local or systemic reactions in recipients. The reactions noted with the anthrax and botulinum vaccines are not unique. The tetanus-diphtheria vaccine is a toxoid vaccine, and is employed worldwide without evidence of inducing chronic medical conditions. The "antigenic load" injected into service members is considerable; an even larger volume of antigens was given (up to 75 cc) to employees at Fort Detrick, Maryland. These people were studied over a period of 15 years and no evidence of im mune-associated illness was identified. No other chronic disease has been attributed to vaccine use.

The swine flu episode of the mid-seventies caused large numbers of Americans to receive a new antigenic strain of influenza virus. Over 40 million people received the vaccine. Many of these recipients claimed that the vaccine initiated rheumatoid arthritis or exacerbated their arthritis. Others claimed to have developed neurological complications from the vaccine. However, several prospective studies demonstrated that there was no association between the vaccine administration and the claimants' arthritic conditions (Herron et al., 1979; Kurland et al., 1984). Conflicting data have been presented regarding neurological complications, but the best epidemiological data, from military records, show no increase in the incidence of Guillain-Barré syndrome.

Most or all of the claims for both rheumatic diseases and Guillain-Barré syndrome seem to have been a result of coincidences that were wrongly interpreted to be causal. The U.S. Government did establish a fund to settle claims, but this was done in order to avoid legal expenses rather than because of a confirmed association between exposure and complications.

The introduction of other vaccines in the last 30 years has been associated with similar examples of coincidences, such as a concern about neurological disease after use of a measles vaccine. One striking exception to this was the polio vaccine. The attenuated living strains have caused paralytic disease in a few recipients or persons infected from a vaccine recipient. Also, a "killed" polio vaccine that had been incompletely treated caused a form of polio. These are examples of disease that clearly can be attributed to the vaccine. We have no evidence that vaccines in general cause the non-specific complaints associated with service during Operation Desert Storm.

Pyridostigmine Bromide

Pyridostigmine bromide (PB) is a drug that belongs to the group of agents classified as anticholinesterases (AChE) that bind reversibly with acetylcholinesterase. This allows the temporary and partial buildup of acetylcholine, which may allow continuous stimulation of cholinergic receptors throughout the central and peripheral nervous system. This pharmacological action has been taken advantage of in the protection of military personnel from the effects of organophosphate toxic gases; these agents bind *irreversibly* with AChE causing life-threatening complications. PB can compete for binding sites and allow escape of AChE to permit more controlled transmission of nerve impulses. Anti-AChE agents are not new drugs. The first drug in this group, Physostigmine, was isolated in 1864. PB has been used for decades to treat patients with myasthenia gravis. (The dose employed is 360 mg to 6,000 mg daily.) There is a great deal of pharmacological data, therefore, about the use of this drug.

Some persons have claimed, however, that the dose recommended for use in military personnel in the war against Iraq (30 mg three times a day) had not been adequately tested in persons who have no diseases such as myasthenia gravis. Certain medical conditions can be made worse by anti-AChE agents. Thus, persons with asthma, coronary artery disease, or cardiac dysrhythmias (especially bradycardia) may have a worsening of their condition, and those who are sensitive to the drug may develop anaphylactic shock. These conditions occur promptly after an overdose of the drug; discontinuation of the drug and the administration of atropine lead to rapid recovery in most people. PB is poorly absorbed from the gastrointestinal tract. The bioavailability is 8 percent to 29 percent of ingested dose. It is 70 percent to 90 percent eliminated unchanged in the urine with the half-life of 3.7 hours. The maximum plasma concentration is reached in 1.7 hours. There is minimal penetration of the blood-brain barrier by this drug.

The side effects of PB include those expected from stimulation of the peripheral parasympathetic nervous system, including nausea, vomiting, diarrhea, abdominal cramps, increased peristalsis, increased salivation, bronchial secretions, miosis, and diaphoresis. Skeletal neuromuscular junctions also are stimulated; the effects involve striated muscle groups—muscle cramps, fasciculation, and weakness. The bromide radical can cause skin rashes which subside when the drug is stopped. There have been no documented long-term side effects of the drug. No effects on pregnancy are known, but there is no evidence to suggest any adverse effects. All of the side effects noted above have been reported in PG military personnel taking PB for varying periods, including up to 50 percent in the U.S. Army Medical Research Institute of Chemical Defense (USAMRICD) study, 38 percent in flight crews, and 48 percent of those seen in health care facilities in the theater of operation. Gastrointestinal symptoms were the most common complaint.

The frequency of these complaints was surprising in light of the few complaints among volunteers who took the same dose, but under more controlled experimental conditions. A possible explanation of these effects was the Stress of being in a hot desert environment and under the threats common to battlegrounds. A study of a small number of volunteers in a desert environment failed to show any difference in symptoms while taking PB versus a placebo (Cook et al., 1992). PB does raise body temperature slightly because it decreases blood flow to the skin, thus limiting heat loss by convection. Offsetting this effect is the increased sweating that occurs as a consequence of PB. In the volunteer study, the slight increase in temperature did not affect exercise tolerance in the heated chamber.

Other explanations for a possible increase in symptoms following PB ingestion have been raised by staff of the Senate Committee on Veterans Affairs. First, the reactions of women may differ from those of men, especially if they are on birth control pills; the effects of PB on women have not been studied. Second, the troops were not screened for those conditions that are contraindications to use of PB, including asthma, peptic ulcer disease, liver disease, kidney disease, or hypersensitivity to PB, though predeployment medical examinations should assume that these conditions, other than sensitivity, were present in few of the troops on active duty. A third hypothesis is a possible synergistic reaction between PB, the pesticides, the insect repellent-impregnated clothing used by the troops, or all of these. It has been known for many years that the simultaneous or sequential administration of two anti-AChE drugs would have an additive or even a synergistic effect. The staff of the Senate Committee cited recent studies in cockroaches, in which a combination of the "pesticide" DEET (actually an insect repellent) and PB was reported to be 10 times as toxic as DEET alone. Several pesticides in low doses are not toxic to most humans, but are effective against insects. Robbins and Cherniack (1986) have reported that DEET is only partially absorbed through the skin of humans and is rapidly but not completely excreted. DEET impairs mammalian biochemical pathways (reversibly inhibiting the urea cycle) and can block lactate-dependent synthesis of glucose (Heick et al., 1988; Brini and Tremblay, 1991).

Pesticides such as permethrin (i.e., synthetic pyrethoids) modify the ionic permeability of nerve membranes and produce a neuroexcitatory toxic response (Casida et al., 1983; Vijverberg and van den Berchen, 1990). They have been shown to act in a stereospecific fashion, that is, in a fashion directly dependent upon the structural conformation of the pesticides, on sodium channels in nerve membranes (Eells et al., 1992). Permethrin has also been found to inhibit calcium-dependent ATP-ase enzyme activity in cells from the central nervous system (Kodavanti et al., 1993).

Inhaled pesticides plus PB conceivably could have synergistic effects, but such effects would be immediately obvious, as was true for the combination that killed the cockroaches. The drugs do not persist in the body, and the IOM committee knows of no pharmacological reason why they should have any long-term effect.

Other medications could possibly increase the risk of side effects of PB. Those drugs would include the beta-blockers used for treating hypertension. This combination could cause a further reduction in cardiac output and blood pressure. In rare persons, there could be bronchial constriction. A combination of PB with medications that cause vasodilation, for example calcium channel blockers, or direct-acting vasodilators in circumstances of poor hydration, could lead to lightheaded feelings or syncope. Antimalarial medications in combination with PB could lead to diarrhea. Quinidine and PB could induce heart block, but the former is not used routinely for malaria prophylaxis or treatment. All these possible drug interactions (and others not mentioned) cause acute and short-lived problems. There is no evidence of any chronic effect.

In summary, PB is a well-studied medication belonging to a class of drugs about which extensive knowledge exists. The DSB Task Force recommended doing a study of the effects of the drug and its metabolites to determine whether they cause long-term effects. The DSB Task Force believed that this was necessary because PB can prevent or ameliorate serious consequences of chemical warfare and must therefore be kept in the military's pharmacopoeia. It seems unlikely that these studies will be revealing, because so much information is available already, and the drug is excreted essentially unchanged.

Depleted Uranium

Daxon (1994) has reported that:

> Natural uranium is composed of three radioactive isotopes: U-238 (99.3 percent by weight), U-235 (0.7 percent), and U-234 (0.006 percent). The depleted uranium (DU) used by DoD is a by-product of the uranium enrichment process that increases the concentration of U-235 to levels suitable for nuclear power and nuclear weapons. The uranium that remains is "depleted" in both U-235 and U-234 and typically contains 0.2 percent of U-235 and 0.001 percent of U-234. Because the radioactive decay rate of U-235 and especially of U-234 is so much higher than U-238, this decrease reduces the radioactivity of DU by approximately 50 percent when compared to natural uranium. The specific activity of natural uranium is 0.7 μCi/g while DU is 0.4 μCi/g. DU is used by DoD in antitank munitions and in tank armor because of its high density and pyrophoric properties.

Intact DU munitions and armor radiation exposure is minimal and within accepted standards. A series of studies conducted by the DoD quantified the radiation exposure received by personnel during the transportation, storage, and use of DU-containing systems. Studies have shown that, with the exception of warehouses where large quantities of DU munitions were stored, the estimated annual exposure did not exceed the current standard of 100 mrem/year for the general population. Where this limit might be exceeded, standard radiation protection programs are in place (Daxon, 1994).

DU can enter the body on the battle field as a result of fires involving DU munitions, use of DU munitions, or working in a vehicle or other space con taminated with DU. Daxon (1994) continues: "In general, only a small fraction (less than 1 percent) of DU particulates from storage or tanks fires were respirable, and more than 90 percent of the respirable particulates were insoluble. When a DU munition strikes an armored target, the fraction of particulates generated that are respirable ranges from 50 percent to 90 percent. Approximately 17 percent to 48 percent of the respirable particles are soluble in lung fluid."

The potential for inhaled DU particles to exceed current safety standards exists only inside vehicles when they are penetrated by DU munitions. This was shown from estimates of simulated bulk storage fires, test fires involving vehicles with DU munitions, and tests in which DU munitions struck armored vehicles. The Persian Gulf experience showed that DU can reach internal body sites through wound contamination and the injection of DU fragments.

DU inside the body presents both radiological and toxicological risks. Irreparable kidney damage has been shown in studies of injected or inhaled uranium salts. The toxic level for uranium in the kidney for single exposures is 1–3 μg of uranium per gram of kidney (Kearsley and Daxon, 1993). However, there is considerable uncertainty regarding the toxicity of long-term exposure to uranium.

The toxicological hazards of DU inhalation and ingestion are probably more significant than the radiological hazards if the uranium compounds internalized are soluble. For insoluble compounds, the ingestion hazards (both radiological and toxicological) are minimal because the majority of the ingested compounds are rapidly eliminated from the body. The risks associated with the inhalation of insoluble compounds are primarily radiological and are determined by the total radiation exposure to the body. The radiological and toxicological hazards associated with long-term exposure to imbedded fragments are uncertain. There are no known studies of the long-term effects of uranium metal implanted in tissues.

During the Persian Gulf War, few personnel were exposed to DU. A friendly fire incident wounded 35 U.S. soldiers, of whom 22 were suspected to have retained DU fragments (Daxon, 1993). Soldiers (27) from the 144th Supply and Service Company involved in fighting fires, vehicle recovery, and cleaning of the 29 tanks damaged by DU munitions were potentially exposed. There were 32 others that had a chance of exposure. DU rounds were left on the battlefield.

A five-year follow-up policy has been developed for the 22 soldiers suspected of having retained DU particles and for all others suspected of being exposed to DU (Keogh, 1993). The Armed Forces Radiobiology Research Institute (AFRRI) reviewed this policy and found that there were sufficient uncertainties with the potential chronic effects to warrant long-term follow-up of veterans with fragments and to conduct research. The Department of De fense and the Department of Veterans Affairs are conducting the recommended patient review and the Department of Defense is initiating AFRRI-recommended research.

Environmental Research Centers

In January 1994 the VA announced a program to establish centers for basic and clinical science studies of environmental hazards. Up to $500,000 per year would be provided for up to five years of support for centers to engage in basic research on environmental health effects, with special emphasis on the diagnosis and treatment of medical problems currently being reported by the PGW veterans. An additional $100,000 will be available for equipment in the first year. The VA is especially interested in new initiatives that complement current activities, and has suggested that interorganizational agreements and scientific affiliations are encouraged if they are justified and set up properly. Links with non-VA researchers are allowed.

As of May 13, 1994, the VA Central Office reported that a group of six "distinguished and internationally renowned scientists was selected to be the ad hoc Scientific Review Committee for the proposals." They were selected on their reputation as "outstanding in the field of environmental science." The committee was to operate much like an NIH study section group; it was to "exclusively make judgment on the scientific quality of each proposal."

These environmental research centers were established in July 1994, in the Veterans Affairs Medical Centers in Boston, Massachusetts; East Orange, New Jersey; and Portland, Oregon. The environmental centers are expected to be fully funded by October 1, 1994. The grants are for five years and there will be a mid-point review conducted by a panel of experts other than the ad hoc committee.

Constituting the ad hoc committee to review proposals and having a mid-term review are excellent ideas; however, the halfway point for a review may come too late. This committee recommends a review by an advisory committee at six months and then every year. The VA should examine how the entire problem can be investigated, and should provide a sufficient degree of central evaluation and advice. Possibly, an external advisory committee could be established, and collaboration with qualified investigators and other federal and non-federal agencies more strongly encouraged.

Review should ensure that appropriate infrastructures will be in place and that funding will support new initiatives and not simply fund current projects. Limiting the non-recurring instrumentation expenditures to $100,000 will surely lead to core laboratories with limited or out-moded testing capabilities.

There is a concern about funding levels for these studies and whether there is going to be sufficient funding to keep these studies going.

References

AFIP (Armed Forces Institute of Pathology). 1993. Kuwait Persian Gulf Registry. Summary Statement by Victor Kalasinsky, data table by Jose Centeno.

APA (American Psychological Association). 1987. DSM-III-R: Diagnostic and Statistical Manual of Mental Disorders, 3rd ed. Washington, D.C.: APA.

Bender AP, Williams AN, Johnson RA, Jagger HG. 1990. Appropriate public health responses to clusters: The art of being responsibly responsive. American Journal of Epidemiology 132 (Suppl 1):S48–S52.

Berg W. 1994. Post-Persian Gulf Medical Findings: Naval Mobile Construction Battalion 24. Presentation to the IOM Committee to Review Health Consequences of Service during the Persian Gulf War. Washington, D.C., January 1994, and Presentation to NIH Technology Assessment Workshop Panel on the Persian Gulf Experience and Health, Bethesda, Md., April 1994.

Blanck R. 1994. Trip Report of Meetings with Coalition Members of Operation Desert Storm/Desert Shield Concerning Reports of Low-Level Chemical Warfare Agent Detection and Health of Their Forces. Memo to the Army Surgeon General from Major General Ronald Blanck.

Brini CM, Tremblay GC. 1991. Reversible inhibition of the urea cycle and gluconeogenesis by N, N-diethyl-m-toluamide. Biochemical and Biophysical Research Communications 179 (3):1264–1268.

Caldwell GG. 1990. Twenty-two years of cancer cluster investigations at the Centers for Disease Control. American Journal of Epidemiology 132(Suppl 1):S43–S47.

Casida JE, Gammon DW, Glickman AH. 1983. Mechanisms of selective action of pyrethroid insecticides. Annual Review of Pharmacology and Toxicology 23:413–438.

Cook JE, Kolka MA. Wenger CB. 1992. Chronic pyridostigmine bromide administration: Side effects among soldiers working in a desert environment. Military Medicine 157(5):250–254.

Cotton P. 1992. Gulf War symptoms remain puzzling. Journal of the American Medical Association 268(19):2619.

CRS (Congressional Research Service). 1992. Iraq-Kuwait crisis: A chronology of events , July 17, 1990–December 23, 1991. Washington, D.C.: The Library of Congress.

Cutler JJ, Parker GS, Rosen 5, Prenney B, Healey R, Caldwell GG. 1986. Childhood leukemia in Woburn, Massachusetts. Public Health Reports 101(2):201–205.

Daxon, EG. 1993. Protocol for Monitoring Gulf War Veterans with Imbedded Fragments of Depleted Uranium. AFRRI Technical Report 93-2. Bethesda, Md.: Armed Forces Radiobiology Research Institute.

Daxon, EG. 1994. DU Exposures during the Persian Gulf War. Presentation to NIH Technology Assessment Workshop Panel on the Persian Gulf Experience and Health, Bethesda, Md., April 1994.

DeFraites, RF, Wanat ER, Norwood AE, William S, Cowan D, Callahan T. Investigation of a Suspected Outbreak of an Unknown Disease among Veterans of Operation Desert Shield/ Storm, 123d Army Reserve Command, Fort Benjamin Harrison, Indiana, April 1992. Washington, D.C.: Walter Reed Army Institute of Research.

DSB (Defense Science Board). 1994. Final Report: Defense Science Board Task Force on Persian Gulf War Health Effects. Washington, D.C.: Office of the Under Secretary of Defense for Acquisition and Technology.

Eells JT, Bandettini PA, Holman PA, Propp JM. 1992. Pyrethroid insecticide-induced alterations in mammalian synaptic membrane potential. Journal of Pharmacology and Experimental Therapeutics 262(3):1173–1181.

EPA (Environmental Protection Agency). 1991. Kuwait Oil Fires: Interagency Interim Report. Washington, D.C.: EPA.

Farrar JT. 1994. Under Secretary for Health Information Letter. Medical Care Programs for Persian Gulf Veterans, Including Comprehensive Clinical Examination Protocol. June 17, 1994. Washington, D.C.

GAO (U.S. General Accounting Office). 1994. Operation Desert Storm: Questions remain on possible exposure to reproductive toxicants. Washington, D.C.: GAO.

Gray G. 1994. Epidemiologic Studies of Morbidity among Gulf War Veterans: A Search for Etiologic Agents and Risk Factors. A presentation to the IOM Committee to Review Health Consequences of Service during the Persian Gulf War, Washington, D.C., August 1994.

Heick HMC, Peterson RG, Dalpe-Scott M, Qureshi IA. 1988. Insect repellent, *N, N*-Diethyl-*m*-toluamide, effect on ammonia metabolism. Pediatrics 82(3):373–376.

Herron A, Dettleff G, Hixon B, Brandwin L, Ortbals D, Hornick R, Hahn B. 1979. Influenza vaccination in patients with rheumatic diseases: Safety and efficacy. Journal of the American Medical Association 242(1):53–56.

Kearsley EE, Daxon EG. 1993. Depleted Uranium: Questions and Answers. AFRRI Technical Report 93-3. Bethesda, Md.: Armed Forces Radiobiology Research Institute. [Note: This report has not been cleared for public release].

Keogh JP. 1993. Proposal to the Department of Veterans Affairs Program for Follow-up Monitoring of Gulf War Veterans with Imbedded Fragments of Depleted Uranium. Baltimore, Md.: Baltimore Veterans Affairs Medical Center.

Kodavanti PRS, Mundy WR, Tilson HA, Harry GJ. 1993. Effects of selected neuroactive chemicals on calcium transporting systems in rat cerebellum and on survival of cerebellar granule cells. Fundamental and Applied Toxicology 21:308–316.

Kreutzer RD, Grogl M, Neva FA, Fryauff DJ, Magill AJ, Aleman-Munoz MM. 1993. Identification and genetic comparison of leishmanial parasites causing viscerotropic and cutaneous disease in soldiers returning from Operation Desert Storm. American Journal of Tropical Medicine 49(3):357–363.

Kurland LT, Molgaard CA, Kurland EM, Erdtmann FJ, Stebbing GT. 1984. Lack of association of swine flu vaccine and rheumatoid arthritis. Mayo Clinic Proceedings (59):816–821.

Lesho EP. 1991. Leishmaniasis: Another threat to Persian Gulf veterans. Postgraduate Medicine 90:213–217.

Magill AJ. 1994. Leishmaniasis as a Potential Cause of Gulf War-Related Illnesses. Presentation to the IOM Committee to Review Health Consequences of Service during the Persian Gulf War, Washington, D.C., August 1994.

Magill AJ, Grögl M, Gasser RA, Sun W, Oster CN. 1993. Visceral infection caused by *Leishmania tropica* in veterans of Operation Desert Storm. New England Journal of Medicine 328 (19):1383–1387.

Marlowe DH, Martin JA, Gifford RK. 1990. Observations and Initial Findings of the WRAIR Stress Evaluation Team: Operation Desert Shield: 22 September–6 October 90. Washington. D.C.: Walter Reed Army Institute of Research.

Mattison DR. 1994. A Framework for Diagnosis: Reproductive and Developmental Toxicity. Presentation to NIH Technology Assessment Workshop Panel on the Persian Gulf Experience and Health, Bethesda, Md., April 1994.

Mississippi State Department of Health. 1994. Mississippi State Department of Health Preliminary Findings on Children of Gulf War Vets. Health Communications and Public Relations . Jackson, Mississippi. April 27, 1994.

MMWR (Morbidity and Mortality Weekly Report). 1992. Viscerotropic leishmaniasis in persons returning from Operation Desert Storm—1990–1991. MMWR 41(8):131–134.

NIH Technology Assessment Workshop Panel. 1994. The Persian Gulf experience and health. Journal of the American Medical Association 272(5):391–396.

Norton SA, Frankenburg S, Klaus SN. 1992. Cutaneous leishmaniasis acquired during military service in the Middle East. Archives of Dermatology 128:83–87.

NRC (National Research Council), Committee on Toxicology. 1994. Health Effects of Permethrin-Impregnated Army Battle-Dress Uniforms. Washington, D.C.: National Academy Press.

O'Donnell FL. 1994. Environmental Conditions in Saudi Arabia. Presentation to NIH Technology Assessment Workshop Panel on the Persian Gulf Experience and Health, Bethesda, Md., April 1994.

Ohl CA, Hyams KC, Malone JD, Oldfield E, III. 1993. Leishmaniasis among Desert Storm veterans: A diagnostic and therapeutic dilemma. Military Medicine 158(11):726–729.

PGVCB (Persian Gulf Veterans Coordinating Board). 1994. Summary of the Issues Impacting upon the Health of Persian Gulf Veterans, Version 3.0. Washington, D.C.: Support Office of the Persian Gulf Veterans Coordinating Board.

Rappaport SM. 1993. Threshold limit values, permissible exposure limits and feasibility: The bases for exposure limits in the United States. American Journal of Industrial Medicine 23:683–694.

Rashti MAS, Panah HY, Mohamadi HS, Jedari M. 1992. Susceptibility of *Phlebotomus papatasi* to DDT in some foci of cutaneous leishmaniasis in Iran. Journal of the American Mosquito Control Association 8(1):99–100.

Richards AL, Hyams KC, Merrell BR, Dasch GA, Woody JN, Ksiazek TG, LeDuc JW, Watts DM. 1991. Medical aspects of Operation Desert Storm [letter]. New England Journal of Medicine 325(13):970.

Richards AL, Malone JD, Sheris S, Weddle JR, Rossi CA, Ksiazek TG, LeDuc JW, Dasch GA, Hyams KC. 1993. Arbovirus and rickettsial infections among combat troops during Operation Desert Shield/Desert Storm [letter]. Journal of Infectious Diseases 168:1080–1081.

Riley EB. 1992. Operation Desert Shield/Desert Storm. History of Participation by the U.S. Army Environmental Hygiene Agency, Aberdeen Proving Ground, Maryland (7 August 1990–31 December 1991). Aberdeen Proving Ground, Md.: USAEHA.

Robbins PJ, Cherniack MG. 1986. Review of the biodistribution and toxicity of the insect repellent *N, N*-Diethyl-*m*-toluamide (DEET). Journal of Toxicology and Environmental Health 18:503–525.

Rothman KJ. 1990. A sobering start for the cluster busters' conference. American Journal of Epidemiology 132 (Suppl 1):S6–S13.

Sanford JP. 1994. Gulf War Syndrome: Proposed Provisional Case Definition. Memo to Major General Ronald Blanck from Jay P. Sanford, M.D.

Scotti JR, Beach BK, Northrop LME, Forsyth JP, Rode CA, Szymanski LA, Beeler LL, Cornell KM. 1993. An Investigation of the Effects of Involvement in Operation Desert Storm: Psychological Distress in the Veteran, Spouse, and Children. Pre sented at the annual convention of the Association for the Advancement of Behavior Therapy, November 1993, Atlanta, Georgia.

Sloan P, Arsenault L, Hilsenroth M, Harvill L. Unpublished (a). Measures of acute post-traumatic stress in Persian Gulf War veterans . Mountain Home, Tn., VAMC.

Sloan P. Arsenault L, Hilsenroth M, Harvill L, Handler L. Unpublished (b). Rorschach measures of post-traumatic stress in Persian Gulf War veterans. Mountain Home, Tn., VAMC.

Sutker PB, Uddo M, Brailey K, Allain AN. 1993. War-zone trauma and stress-related symptoms in Operation Desert Shield/Storm (ODS) returnees. Journal of Social Issues 49(4):33–49.

Sutker PB, Uddo M, Brailey K, Allain AN, Errera P. 1994a. Psychological symptoms and psychiatric diagnoses in Operation Desert Storm troops serving graves registration duty. Journal of Traumatic Stress 7(2):159–171.

Sutker PB, Uddo M, Brailey K, Vasterling JJ, Errera P. 1994b. Psychopathology in war-zone deployed and nondeployed Operation Desert Storm troops assigned graves registration duties. Journal of Abnormal Psychology 103(2):383–390.

USAEHA (U.S. Army Environmental Hygiene Agency). 1992. Interim Kuwait Oil Fire Health Risk Assessment, No. 39-26-L192-91, 5 May–15 September 1991. Aberdeen Proving Ground, Md.: USAEHA.

USAEHA. 1994a. Final Report—Kuwait Oil Fire Health Risk Assessment, No. 39-26-L192-91, 5 May–3 December 1991. Aberdeen Proving Ground, Md.: USAEHA.

USAEHA. 1994b. Biological Surveillance Initiative. Appendix F of Final Report Kuwait Oil Fire Health Risk Assessment, No. 39-26-L192-91, 5 May–3 December 1991. Aberdeen Proving Ground, Md.: USAEHA.

VA (Department of Veterans Affairs). 1994. Update on Persian Gulf Research, Prepared by the Department of Veterans Affairs, Office of Research and Development, Medical Research Service. In collaboration with the Persian Gulf Interagency Research Coordinating Council. September 19, 1994. Washington, D.C.: VA Central Office.

VA. 1992a. VA Manual. M-10, Part III, Chapter 2. Washington, D.C.

VA. 1992b. Returning Persian Gulf Troops: First Year Findings. West Haven Ct.: VA Northeast Program Evaluation Center.

Vijverberg HPM, van den Berchen J. 1990. Neurotoxicological effects and the mode of action of pyrethroid insecticides. Critical Reviews in Toxicology 21(2):105–126.

Wolfe J, Brown PJ, Kelley JM. 1993. Reassessing war stress. Exposure and the Persian Gulf War. Journal of Social Issues 49(4):15–31.

A

Putative Outcomes and Exposures

PUTATIVE OUTCOMES

Adverse pregnancy outcomes
Amenorrhea
Cancer
Chronic fatigue syndrome
Chronic respiratory effects
Depression or post-traumatic stress disorder
Excess or early mortality
Infertility
Joint pain
Memory loss
Multiple chemical sensitivities
"Mystery Illness," "Gulf War Syndrome"

PUTATIVE EXPOSURES

Chemical warfare, biological warfare
Depleted uranium
Infectious tropical diseases—such as leishmaniasis
Microwaves
Multiple chemical exposures

Oil well fires
Pesticides
Petrochemicals—diesel fuels/tent heaters
Physical strain
Pyridostigmine
Rape or sexual harassment
Stress
Vaccination, inoculations, medications

B

Invited Presentations

Mr. Fred Ambrose, Defense Intelligence Agency, Washington, D.C.

Dr. Drue Barrett, Centers for Disease Control and Prevention, Atlanta, Georgia

CAPT William Berg, MC, Navy Environmental and Preventive Medicine Unit No. 2, Norfolk, Virginia

MAJ Stephen Berté, U.S. Army Medical Material Development Activity, Fort Detrick, Maryland

Dr. Sal Bosco, Defense Science Board Task Force on Chemical Weapons, Washington, D.C.

COL Frank Cox, Defense Science Board Task Force on Chemical Weapons, Washington, D.C.

LTC Robert DeFraites, MC, Walter Reed Army Institute of Research, Washington, D.C.

Mr. Layne Drash, VA Central Office, Washington, D.C.

LTC Edward Eitzen, MC, U.S. Army Medical Research Institute of Infectious Diseases, Frederick, Maryland

CDR Gregory C. Gray, MC, Naval Health Research Center, San Diego, California

Mr. Don Hakenson, U.S. Army Joint Services Environmental Support Group, Fort Belvoir, Virginia

Dr. Rogene Henderson, National Academy of Sciences, Committee on Toxicology, Washington, D.C.

COL Charles G. Hurst, MC, U.S. Army Medical Research Institute of Chemical Defense, Aberdeen Proving Ground, Maryland

Dr. Han Kang, VA Central Office, Washington, D.C.

MAJ William Legg, U.S. Army Environmental Hygiene Agency, Aberdeen Proving Ground, Maryland

LTC Alan Magill, MC, Walter Reed Army Institute of Research, Washington, D.C.

Dr. Frances Murphy, VA Central Office, Washington, D.C.

Dr. Neil Otchin, VA Central Office, Washington, D.C.

LTC Terry Rauch, MC, Office of Assistant Secretary of Defense, Washington, D.C.

Dr. Fred Sidell, U.S. Army Medical Research Institute of Chemical Defense, Aberdeen Proving Ground, Maryland

Dr. Robert Ursano, Uniformed Services University of the Health Sciences, Bethesda, Maryland

Dr. Bernard Wagner, National Academy of Sciences, Committee on Toxicology, Washington, D.C.

Dr. Diana Zuckerman, staff to Senate Veterans Affairs Committee, Washington, D.C.

C

Portions of PL 102-25, PL 102-190, and PL 102-585

PL 102-25 Persian Gulf Service and PTSD

SEC. 335 REPORTS BY SECRETARY OF DEFENSE AND SECRETARY OF VETERANS AFFAIRS CONCERNING SERVICES TO TREAT POST-TRAUMATIC STRESS DISORDER

(a) IN GENERAL.—The Secretary of Defense and the Secretary of Veterans Affairs shall each submit to Congress two reports containing, with respect to their respective Departments, the following:

(1) An assessment of the need for rehabilitative services for members of the Armed Forces participating in the Operation Desert Storm who experience post-traumatic stress disorder.

(2) A description of the available programs and resources to meet those needs.

(3) The specific plans of that Secretary for treatment of members experiencing post-traumatic stress disorder, particularly with respect to any specific needs of members of reserve components.

(4) An assessment of needs for additional resources necessary in order to carry out such plans.

(5) A description of plans to coordinate treatment services for post-traumatic stress disorder with the other Department.

(b) TIMES FOR SUBMISSION OF REPORTS.—The first report by each of the Secretaries shall be submitted not later than 90 days after the date of the enactment of this Act, and the second report by each of the Secretaries shall be submitted a year later.

PL 102-190 DoD to Establish PG Registry

SEC. 734 REGISTRY OF MEMBERS OF THE ARMED FORCES EXPOSED TO FUMES OF BURNING OIL IN CONNECTION WITH OPERATION DESERT STORM.

(a) ESTABLISHMENT OF REGISTRY.—The Secretary of Defense shall establish and maintain a special record relating to members of the Armed Forces who, as determined by the Secretary, were exposed to the fumes of burning oil in the Operation Desert Storm theater of operations during the Persian Gulf conflict. The Secretary shall establish the Registry with the advice of an independent scientific organization.

(b) CONTENTS OF REGISTRY.—The Registry shall include—

(1) a list containing the name of each member referred to in subsection (a); and

(2) a description of the circumstances of each exposure of that member to the fumes of burning oil as described in subsection (a), including the length of time of the exposure.

(C) REPORTING REQUIREMENT RELATING TO EXPOSURE STUDIES.—The Secretary shall submit to Congress each year, at or about the time that the President's budget is submitted that year under section 1105 of title 31, United States Code, a report regarding—

(1) the results of all on-going studies on the members referred to in subsection (a) to determine the health consequences (including any short or long-term consequences) of the exposure of such members to the fumes of burning oil; and

(2) the need for additional studies relating to the exposure of such members to such fumes.

(d) MEDICAL EXAMINATION.—Upon the request of any member listed in the registry, the Secretary of the military department concerned shall, if medically appropriate, furnish a pulmonary function examination and chest x-ray to such person.

(e) EFFECTIVE DATE.—The Secretary shall establish the Registry not later that 180 days after the date of the enactment of this Act.

(f) DEFINITIONS.—For Purposes of this section:

(1) The term "Operation Desert Storm" has the meaning given such term in section 3(1) of the Persian Gulf Conflict Supplemental Authorization and

Personnel Benefits Act of 1991 (Public Law 102-25; 105 Stat. 77; 10 U.S.C. 101 note).

(2) The term "Persian Gulf conflict" has the meaning given such term in section 3(3) of such Act.

PL 102-585 Persian Gulf War Veterans' Health Status

SEC. 702. PERSIAN GULF WAR VETERANS HEALTH REGISTRY.

(a) ESTABLISHMENT OF REGISTRY.—The Secretary of Veterans Affairs shall establish and maintain a special record to be known as the "Persian Gulf War Veterans Health Registry" (in this section referred to as the "Registry").

(b) CONTENTS OF REGISTRY.—Except as provided in subsection (c), the Registry shall include the following information:

(1) A list containing the name of each individual who served as a member of the Armed Forces in the Persian Gulf theater of operations during the Persian Gulf War and who—

(A) applies for care or services from the Department of Veterans Affairs under chapter 17 of title 38, United States Code;

(B) files a claim for compensation under chapter 11 of such title on the basis of any disability which may be associated with such service;

(C) dies and is survived by a spouse, child, or parent who files a claim for dependency and indemnity compensation under chapter 13 of such title on the basis of such service;

(D) requests from the Department a health examination under section 703; or

(E) receives from the Department of Defense a health examination similar to the health examination referred to in subparagraph (D) and requests inclusion in the Registry.

(2) Relevant medical data relating to the health status of, and other information that the Secretary considers relevant and appropriate with respect to, each individual described in paragraph (1) who— (A) grants to the Secretary permission to include such information in the Registry; or

(B) at the time the individual is listed in the Registry, is deceased.

(c) INDIVIDUALS SUBMITTING CLAIMS OR MAKING REQUESTS BEFORE DATE OF ENACTMENT.—If in the case of an individual described in subsection (b)(1) the application, claim, or request referred to in such sub section was submitted, filed, or made, before the date of the enactment of this Act, the Secretary shall, to the extent feasible, include in the Registry such individual's name and the data and information, if any, described in subsection (b)(2) relating to the individual.

(d) DEPARTMENT OF DEFENSE INFORMATION.—The Secretary of Defense shall furnish to the Secretary of Veterans Affairs such information maintained by the Department of Defense as the Secretary of Veterans Affairs considers necessary to establish and maintain the Registry.

(e) RELATION TO DEPARTMENT OF DEFENSE REGISTRY.—The Secretary of Veterans Affairs, in consultation with the Secretary of Defense, shall ensure that information is collected and maintained in the Registry in a manner that permits effective and efficient cross-reference between the Registry and the registry established under section 734 of the National Defense Authorization Act for Fiscal Years 1992 and 1993 (Public Law 102-190; 105 Stat. 1411; 10 U.S.C. 1074 note), as amended by section 704.

(f) ONGOING OUTREACH TO INDIVIDUALS LISTED IN REGISTRY. —The Secretary of Veterans Affairs shall, from time to time, notify individuals listed in the Registry of significant developments in research on the health consequences of military service in the Persian Gulf theater of operations during the Persian Gulf War.

SEC. 703. HEALTH EXAMINATIONS AND COUNSELING FOR VETERANS ELIGIBLE FOR INCLUSION IN CERTAIN HEALTH-RELATED REGISTRIES.

(a) In General.—(1) The Secretary of Veterans Affairs—

(A) shall, upon the request of a veteran described in subsection (b)(1), provide the veteran with a health examination and consultation and counseling with respect to the results of the examination; and

(B) may, upon the request of a veteran described in subsection (b)(2), provide the veteran with such an examination and such consultation and counseling.

(2) The Secretary shall carry out appropriate outreach activities with respect to the provision of any health examinations and consultations and counseling services under paragraph (1).

(b) COVERED VETERANS.—(1) In accordance with subsection (a)(1)(A), the Secretary shall provide an examination, consultation, and counseling under that subsection to any veteran who is eligible for listing or inclusion in the Persian Gulf War Veterans Health Registry established by section 702.

(2) In accordance with subsection (a)(1)(B), the Secretary may provide an examination, consultation, and counseling under that subsection to any veteran

who is eligible for listing or inclusion in any other similar health-related registry administered by the Secretary.

SEC. 704. EXPANSION OF COVERAGE OF PERSIAN GULF REGISTRY.

(a) IN GENERAL.—Subsections (a) and (b) of section 734 of the National Defense Authorization Act for Fiscal Years 1992 and 1993 (Public Law 102-190; 105 Stat. 1411; 10 U.S.C. 1074 note) are amended to read as follows:

"(a) ESTABLISHMENT OF REGISTRY.—The Secretary of Defense shall establish and maintain a special record (in this section referred to as the 'Registry') relating to the following members of the Armed Forces:

"(1) Members who, as determined by the Secretary, were exposed to the fumes of burning oil in the Operation Desert Storm theater of operations during the Persian Gulf conflict.

"(2) Any other members who served in the Operation Desert Storm theater of operations during the Persian Gulf conflict.

"(b) CONTENTS OF REGISTRY.—(1) The Registry shall include—

"(A) with respect to each class of members referred to in each of paragraphs (1) and (2) of subsection (a)—

"(i) a list containing each such member's name and other relevant identifying information with respect to the member; and

"(ii) to the extent that data are available and inclusion of the data is feasible, a description of the circumstances of the member's service during the Persian Gulf conflict, including the locations in the Operation Desert Storm theater of operations in which such service occurred and the atmospheric and other environmental circumstances in such locations at the time of such service; and

"(B) with respect to the members referred to in subsection (a)(1), a description of the circumstances of each exposure of each such member to the fumes of burning oil as described in such subsection (a)(1), including the length of time of the exposure.

"(2) The Secretary shall establish the Registry with the advice of an independent scientific organization."

(b) CONFORMING AMENDMENTS.—(1) Subsection (c)(1) of such section is amended by striking out "subsection (a)" and inserting in lieu thereof "subsection (a)(1)."

(2) Subsection (d) of such section is amended by inserting "pursuant to subsection (a)(1)" after "Registry."

SEC. 706. AGREEMENT WITH NATIONAL ACADEMY OF SCIENCES FOR REVIEW OF HEALTH CONSEQUENCES OF SERVICE DURING THE PERSIAN GULF WAR.

(a) AGREEMENT.—(1) The Secretary of Veterans Affairs and Secretary of Defense jointly shall seek to enter into an agreement with the National Academy of Sciences for the Medical Follow-Up Agency (MFUA) of the Institute of Medicine of the Academy to review existing scientific, medical, and other information on the health consequences of military service in the Persian Gulf theater of operations during the Persian Gulf War.

(2) The agreement shall require MFUA to provide members of veterans organizations and members of the scientific community (including the Director of the Office of Technology Assessment) with the opportunity to comment on the method or methods MFUA proposes to use in conducting the review.

(3) The agreement shall permit MFUA, in conducting the review, to examine and evaluate medical records of individuals who are included in the registries referred to in section 705(d) for purposes that MFUA considers appropriate, including the purpose of identifying illnesses of those individuals.

(4) The Secretary of Veterans Affairs and the Secretary of Defense shall seek to enter into the agreement under this section not later than 180 days after the date of the enactment of this Act.

(b) REPORT.—(1) The agreement under this section shall require the National Academy of Sciences to submit to the committees and secretaries referred to in paragraph (2) a report on the results of the review carried out under the agreement. Such report shall contain the following:

(A) An assessment of the effectiveness of actions taken by the Secretary of Veterans Affairs and the Secretary of Defense to collect and maintain information that is potentially useful for assessing the health consequences of the military service referred to in subsection (a).

(B) Recommendations on means of improving the collection and maintenance of such information.

(C) Recommendations on whether there is sound scientific basis for an epidemiological study or studies on the health consequences of such service, and if the recommendation is that there is sound scientific basis for such a study or studies, the nature of the study or studies.

(2) The committees and secretaries referred to in paragraph (1) are the following:

(A) The Committees on Veterans' Affairs of the Senate and House of Representatives.

(B) The Committees on Armed Services of the Senate and House of Representatives.

(C) The Secretary of Veterans Affairs.

(D) The Secretary of Defense.

(c) FUNDING.—(1) The Secretary of Veterans Affairs and the Secretary of Defense shall make available up to a total of $500,000 in fiscal year 1993, from funds available to the Department of Veterans Affairs and the Department of Defense in that fiscal year, to carry out the review. Any amounts provided by the two departments shall be provided in equal amounts.

(2) If the Secretary of Veterans Affairs and the Secretary of Defense enter into an agreement under subsection (a) with the National Academy of Sciences—

(A) the Secretary of Veterans Affairs shall make available $250,000 in each of fiscal years 1994 through 2003, from amounts available to the Department of Veterans Affairs in each such fiscal year, to the National Academy of Sciences for the general purposes of conducting epidemiological research with respect to military and veterans populations; and

(B) the Secretary of Defense shall make available $250,000 in each of fiscal years 1994 through 2003, from amounts available to the Department of Defense in each such fiscal year, to the National Academy of Sciences for the purposes of carrying out the research referred to in subparagraph (A).

SEC. 707. COORDINATION OF GOVERNMENT ACTIVITIES ON HEALTH-RELATED RESEARCH ON THE PERSIAN GULF WAR.

(a) DESIGNATION OF COORDINATING ORGANIZATION.—The President shall designate, and may redesignate from time to time, the head of an appropriate department or agency of the Federal Government to coordinate all research activities undertaken or funded by the Executive Branch of the Federal Government on the health consequences of military service in the Persian Gulf theater of operations during the Persian Gulf War.

(b) REPORT.—Not later than March 1 of each year, the head of the department or agency designated under subsection (a) shall submit to the Committees on Veterans' Affairs of the Senate and House of Representatives a report on the status and results of all such research activities undertaken or by the Executive Branch of the Federal Government during the previous year.

D

Meetings of the IOM Committee

January 20–21, 1994, Washington, D.C.

February 28–March 1, 1994, Washington, D.C. (public meeting)

April 20–21, 1994, Washington, D.C.

July 14–16, 1994, Irvine, California

August 30–September 1, 1994, Washington, D.C.

Presenters at the public meeting:

Mr. Troy Albuck, Persian Gulf veteran, Barrington, Illinois

Ms. Kelli Albuck, spouse of Troy Albuck, Barrington, Illinois

Ms. Helen Ellis, mother of Persian Gulf veteran, Oakton, Virginia

Mr. Paul Guerrette, Persian Gulf veteran, Petersburg, Virginia

Mr. Richard Haines, Army Reservist, New Albany, Indiana

Mr. Kimo Hollingsworth, Persian Gulf veteran, American Legion, Washington, D.C.

Ms. Mary Lamielle, National Center for Environmental Health Strategies, Vorhees, New Jersey

Ms. Penny Larrisey, spouse of Persian Gulf veteran, Philadelphia, Pennsylvania

Mr. Steve Robertson, Persian Gulf veteran, American Legion, Washington, D.C.

Dr. Herbert Smith, Persian Gulf veteran, Ijamsville, Maryland

Dr. Grace Ziem, Occupational Medicine, Baltimore, Maryland

Written testimony supplied for the public meeting:

Ms. Venus-Valiery Hammack, Persian Gulf veteran, Lowell, Massachusetts

Spouse of Venus-Valiery Hammack, Lowell, Massachusetts

Ms. Evelyn Hazen, U.S. Army (retired), Walla Walla, Washington

Mr. Tad Leeds, Persian Gulf veteran

Ms. Jeanette Martinez, spouse of Persian Gulf veteran, San Antonio, Texas

Dr. Ruth Gordon McGill, San Angelo, Texas

Ms. Janelle Payne, spouse of Persian Gulf veteran, Glendale, Arizona

Mr. Anthony Picou, Jr., Operation Desert Shield/Storm Association, Universal City, Texas

Mr. Nick Roberts, Persian Gulf veteran, Phenix City, Alabama

Mr. Paul Sullivan, Persian Gulf veteran, Decatur, Georgia

MAJ Chris Wilman, U.K. Ministry of Defense, British Embassy, Washington, D.C.

Materials were also received from:

Dr. Rupert Ammann, Fort Collins, Colorado

Mr. Albert Donnay, Baltimore, Maryland

Dr. John Ellis, family member of Persian Gulf veteran, Oakton, Virginia

Mr. Joseph Ellis, Persian Gulf veteran, Gainesville, Florida

Ms. Francis Juanice Fox, family member of Persian Gulf veteran, Phoenix, Arizona

Dr. Kendall Gerdes, Denver, Colorado

Mrs. Vickie Gray, Houston, Texas

Mr. Michael Gray, Houston, Texas

Mr. David Greenleaf, Island Pond, Vermont

Mr. Solomon Jamerson, U.S. Army (retired), Los Angeles, California

Dr. Alexander Karczmar, Hines, Illinois

Dr. Boaz Milner, Allen Park, Michigan

Dr. Joseph Neumann, Mountain Home, Tennessee

Dr. Patricia Olson, staff to Senate Veterans Affairs Committee, Washington, D.C.

Ms. Mary Shears, spouse of Persian Gulf veteran, Cedar Rapids, Iowa

Dr. Donald Stewart, Alfred, New York

Dr. Anne Summers, Athens, Georgia

Mr. Lenny Woodard, Persian Gulf veteran, Texarkana, Arkansas

E

Activities (as of September 1994) Related to Potential Health Consequences of Service in the Persian Gulf

Activity	Organization	Nature of Activity
Boards and Committees		
Persian Gulf Expert Scientific Panel	Office of the Chief Medical Director for Environmental Medicine and Public Health, VA	Provide advice to the VA on diagnosis, treatment and research on PG-related health conditions.
Task Force on Persian Gulf War Health Effects	Defense Science Board, DoD	Report to the Under Secretary of Defense (Acquisition) on review of all available *reports* of detection of chemical agents and toxins during ODS/S and postwar period; and review scientific and medical evidence relating exposure to nerve agents, environmental pollutants, endemic biology and other health hazards (DSB, 1994).
Persian Gulf Veterans Coordinating Board	Secretaries of DoD, HHS, and VA	Ensure interagency coordination of all efforts, separate and joint, in the areas of research, clinical care, and disability determination and compensation for post-ODS/S unexplained illnesses (PGVCB, 1994).
Persian Gulf Interagency Research Coordinating Council	DoD, EPA, HHS, and VA	Coordinate all research activities undertaken or funded by the Executive Branch of the federal government on the health consequences of military service in PG theater; VA appointed as lead agency (PL 102-585, sec. 707).

Activity	Organization	Nature of Activity
NIH Technology Assessment Workshop: The Persian Gulf Experience and Health	Persian Gulf Interagency Research Coordinating Council	Develop a case definition of "mystery illness" and provide a list of recommendations. April 27–29, 1994 (NIH Technology Assessment Workshop Panel, 1994).
Population-Based Activities		
Registry of unit locations	Environmental Support Group, Dept. of the Army	Database that identifies the daily location of PG units.
Health-Outcomes-Based Activities—Completed or Well Underway		
Constructing a Case Definition		
Working Group on Unexplained Illnesses	Walter Reed Army Medical Center	Review and analyze medical records of ODS/S veterans with unexplained symptoms to establish a working case definition for post-PG unexplained illnesses.
Outbreak Investigations		
Investigation of a possible outbreak among ODS veterans, Fort Benjamin Harrison, Ind.	Division of Preventive Medicine, WRAIR	Examined and surveyed 79 soldiers with unexplained signs and symptoms.
Post-Persian-Gulf illness reported in Naval Reserve Mobile Construction Battalion 24	Navy Preventive Medicine Unit 2, Dept. of the Navy	Follow-up of members of construction battalion units reporting unexplained signs and symptoms.
VA Health Registry and Clinical Evaluations		
Persian Gulf Health Registry	Environmental Agents Service, VA	Collects data from PG veterans self-referred for examination at VAMC.
Review of Health Registry Data	Environmental Epidemiology Service, VA	Descriptive analysis of registry data.
Persian Gulf Referral Centers	Washington, D.C.; Houston, Texas; and West Los Angeles, Calif.	Local VAMC physicians refer PG veterans for more extensive physical examinations, when needed.
Comprehensive Clinical Evaluation Program	Office of Health Affairs, DoD	Clinical three-phase evaluation of active duty PG veterans and family members with unexplained signs and symptoms.
Mental Health		
Desert Storm Reunion Survey	Boston, Mass., VAMC	Determine impact of combat and noncombat experiences on subsequent patterns of adjustment (NEPEC, 1992; Wolfe et al., 1993).
Neuropsychological and psychological profiles of PG soldiers returning home	Boston, Mass., VAMC	Neuropsychiatric evaluation to diagnose PTSD and anxiety disorders.

Continued

Activity	Organization	Nature of Activity
Development of neuropsychological function norms and assessment of neurotoxin exposure in PGW veterans and controls	Birmingham, Ala., VAMC	Provide basic neuropsychological and environmental exposure database information as core project support for future studies of symptomatic veterans and controls from the PGW.
Early intervention with Appalachian Marine reservists in ODS	Mt. Home, Tenn., VAMC	Debriefing PG veterans on the stresses of deployment and combat-related PTSD (NEPEC, 1992; Sloan et al., unpublished a, b).
Investigation of relation between experience in ODS and postwar adjustment	Clarksburg, W.V., VAMC and Dept. of Psychology, West Virginia University	Investigate the effects that involvement in ODS may have had on veterans, their spouses, or significant others, and their children (Scotti et al., 1993).
Psychological assessment of ODS returnees	New Orleans, La., VAMC	Ongoing debriefing and assessment protocol conducted among troops mobilized in support of the PGW (NEPEC, 1992; Sutker et al., 1993, 1994a, 199b).
Psychological adjustment in ODS/S veterans	Gainesville, Fla., VAMC	Conduct psychological tests to determine if differences existed between PG veterans and controls in terms of overall mental health (NEPEC, 1992).
ODS follow-up survey	Salt Lake City, Utah, VAMC	To elicit VAMC employees' perceptions of ODS activation, deployment, and reintegration experiences.
ODS Outreach Program	Cincinnati, Ohio, VAMC	Explore relation between early life stressors, combat stressors, coping skills and current level of symptomatology.
Other completed VAMC studies		Evaluation of possible psychological consequences of PG service (NEPEC, 1992).
West Haven VAMC ODS report	West Haven, Conn.	(NEPEC, 1992)
The PG Outreach Program at the Little Rock VAMC	Little Rock, Ark.	(NEPEC, 1992)
An Evaluation of Troops Returning from the PG: A Preliminary Report	Providence, R.I.	(NEPEC, 1992)
Coming Home for Good: The ODS Veterans and Family Psychosocial Debriefing Project	Portland, Oreg.	(NEPEC, 1992)

Activity	Organization	Nature of Activity
The Need for Continuing Mental Health Intervention in Soldiers Returning form the PGW: Assessment of Deployed and Non-Deployed Reserve Units from Western Pennsylvania, Eastern Ohio, and West Virginia	Highland Drive, Pa.	(NEPEC, 1992)
PG Veterans Seen Through VA's Readjustment Counseling Service and Impact of the PGW on VA's Provision of Readjustment Counseling	Washington, D.C.	(NEPEC, 1992)
Stress-related surveys of active duty, national guard, and reserve personnel	Dept. of Military Psychology, WRAIR	Assess stresses and psychological and psychosocial impacts of commitment to combat and probable stress consequences, such as posttraumatic and postdeployment stress symptoms and stresses due to return and adjustment.
Leishmaniasis		
Leishmaniasis research	Infectious Disease Section, WRAIR	Clinical assessment of viscerotropic leishmaniasis as a potential cause of some of the unexplained PGW illnesses.
Health-Outcomes-Based Activities—New or Just Beginning		
Reproductive Health		
Children of PG veterans	Jackson, Miss., VAMC, CDC, Miss. State Health Department	Clearinghouse for data on reported birth defects in children of members of Waynesboro, Miss., National Guard.
GAO Birth Defects Report	GAO	Review of reproductive outcomes among children of PG veterans.
Mortality study	Environmental Agents Service, VA	Study of mortality of all PG veterans compared to PG-era veterans.
Health survey	Environmental Agents Service, VA	Study of prevalence of health outcomes in 15,000 PG veterans and 15,000 PG-era veterans.
Iowa survey	National Center for Environmental Health, CDC	Assess prevalence of self-reported adverse health outcomes among Iowa residents who were deployed to the PG during ODS compared to Iowa veterans deployed elsewhere during the same era.

Continued

Activity	Organization	Nature of Activity
Epidemiologic studies of morbidity among PG veterans	Clinical Epidemiology Branch, Naval Health Research Center	1) Cohort study of members of PG and control construction battalions; 2) cohort study of PG veterans and control hospitalization diagnoses; and 3) outcomes of hospitalization for pregnancy among cohorts in study 2.
Exposure-Based Activities		
Environmental		
Air monitoring of oil well fires	U.S. Interagency Air Assessment Team (EPA, HHS, NOAA) and representatives from Coast Guard, DoD, DOE	Assessed pollutants from oil well fires.
Report to Congress: United States Gulf Environmental Technical Assessment (January 27–July 31, 1991)	International cooperative effort coordinated by U.N.; EPA coordinated U.S. activities (PL 102-27, sec. 309)	Coordinated effort of international activities in response to health, atmospheric, and environmental impacts of oil discharge and fires.
Report to Congress on health effects of exposure to burning oil fields	DoD—Depts. of Army, Navy, and Air Force	Results of Army, Navy, and Air Force studies of potential health consequences of exposure to fumes from burning oil.
Environmental toxicology studies	Dept. of Environmental and Toxicologic Pathology, Armed Forces Institute of Pathology	Human autopsy studies; veterinary pathology reports with toxicological results of potentially hazardous PG environmental exposures.
Kuwait Oil Fire Health Risk Assessment	USAEHA	Quantitative assessment of carcinogenic and noncarcinogenic health risks of exposure to oil well fires (USAEHA, 1992; 1994a).
Biologic Surveillance Initiative	USAEHA, Armed Forces Institute of Pathology	Biologic Surveillance Initiative: Surveillance of German-based 11th Armored Calvary (before, during, and after deployment to the PG) (USAEHA 1994b).
Laboratory studies of pesticides	Army Research and Development Command, Dept. of the Army	Proposed activities: USAEHA will study the effects of combined exposure to PB, DEET, and permethrin in rats; South Florida Research Corporation will study the effects of PB in humans (men and women); Duke University will study the delayed reactions in chickens of exposure to DEET, permethrin, and sarin.

Activity	Organization	Nature of Activity
Vaccines and Prophylactic Treatment		
Retrospective survey of PG Troops who received *Clostridium botulinum* toxoid	U.S. Army Medical Materiel Development Activity, Dept. of the Army	Retrospective postcard survey of side-effects in the Marine contingent that received vaccine, Camp Pendleton, Calif., August 1991.
Retrospective studies involving military use of pyridostigmine as pretreatment for nerve agent poisoning	U.S. Army Medical Research Institute of Chemical Defense, Dept. of the Army	Collect safety data for pending New Drug Application to the FDA.
Depleted Uranium		
Monitoring PG veterans with imbedded depleted uranium fragments	Baltimore, Md., VAMC, Dept. of the Army, and University of Maryland	5-year follow-up of soldiers with depleted uranium fragments.
Environmental Centers		
Health effects of environmental exposures during the Persian Gulf War	Boston, Mass., VAMC	Six projects are planned to determine the health effects of environmental exposure to potential hazards, with a particular emphasis on behavioral toxicology, immunotoxicology, cancer epidemiology, and behavioral psychopathology.
Environmental illnesses in PG veterans	The New Jersey Environmental Hazards Research Center, and East Orange, N.J., VAMC	Four projects are planned to gather information about illnesses in PG veterans to develop the most characteristic symptom profiles.
Exposure to environmental, chemical, and biological hazards related to military service	Portland, Ore., VAMC and the Oregon Health Sciences University's Center for Research on Occupational and Environmental Toxicology	Four projects are planned to identify exposures and to define more accurately relations between illnesses in PG veterans and PTSD, or specific environmental, infectious, or chemical warfare exposures.

NOTE: CDC = Centers for Disease Control and Prevention; DoD = Dept. of Defense; DOE = Dept. of Energy; EPA = Environmental Protection Agency; GAO = General Accounting Office; FDA = Food and Drug Administration; HHS = Dept. of Health and Human Services; NIH = National Institutes of Health; NOAA = National Oceanographic and Atmospheric Administration; ODS = Operation Desert Storm; ODS/S = Operation Desert Shield/Desert Storm; PB = pyridostigmine bromide; PG = Persian Gulf; PGVCB = Persian Gulf Veterans Coordinating Board; PGW Persian Gulf War; PL = public law; PTSD posttraumatic stress disorder; USAEHA = U.S. Army Environmental Hygiene Agency; VA = Dept. of Veterans Affairs; VAMC = VA Medical Center; and WRAIR = Walter Reed Army Institute of Research.

F

Timeline of Relevant Events

	1990
August 2	Saddam Hussein invades Kuwait
August 7	Troops begin deployment in Operation Desert Shield
November 8	200,000 troops deployed to join those already in SWA
November 29	UN Resolution 678 authorizing member states to use "all necessary means" to get Iraq out of Kuwait
	1991
January 12	House Joint Resolution 77 authorizes President Bush to use armed force to implement UN Resolution 678
January 14	Resolution signed by President Bush as PL 102-1
January 16	Coalition air forces begin attack of Iraq in Operation Desert Storm
January 20	Iraqis start oil well fires
February 24	Ground war begins
February 28	Persian Gulf War ends
April 3	Interagency Interim Report: Kuwait Oil Fires
June 13	Last troops in ground war return to United States
December 5	PL 102-190 "National Defense Authorization Act" is passed, mandating that DoD create a registry of forces exposed to fumes of burning oil

	1992
April	123rd Army Reserve in Indiana reports illness with unexplained signs and symptoms, investigated by researchers at WRAIR
June 15	Findings of WRAIR investigation released, with no common exposures found among reserves to account for signs and symptoms reported
November 4	PL 102-585 passed, mandating creation of VA Persian Gulf Health Registry, modification of PL 102-190 to include all troops in SWA, asking for NAS review, and OTA review
	1993
May 7	VA Blue Ribbon Panel meeting to discuss "mystery illness"
June 9	Hearing of House Committee on Veterans Affairs Subcommittee on Oversight and Investigation on Health Care Issues of Persian Gulf Veterans
July 29	OTA workshop on Persian Gulf Veterans Health
August 31	President Clinton designated VA to be lead agency for all federally funded Persian Gulf research
October 1	Funding for NAS/IOM review is available
October 16	VA formally chartered the Persian Gulf Expert Scientific Committee (formerly the VA Blue Ribbon Panel)
November 9	Hearing of House Committee on Veterans Affairs on Health Concerns of Persian Gulf Veterans
November 16	Hearing of House Committee on Veterans Affairs Subcommittee on Oversight and Investigation on Health Concerns of Persian Gulf Veterans
November 16	Hearing of Senate Committee on Veterans Affairs on Health Concerns of Persian Gulf Veterans
November 23	Persian Gulf Interagency Coordinating Committee meeting
December 10	As requested by Undersecretary John Deutch, the Defense Science Board Task Force on Chemical Weapons was formed
December 20	Persian Gulf Research Coordinating Council meeting
December 21–22	DSB Task Force on Chemical Weapons meeting
December 21	DSB charter expanded to include Gulf War health effects

	1994
January 10–11	DSB Task Force CBW Panel meeting
January 20–21	IOM Committee meeting
January 21	The formation of the Persian Gulf Veterans Coordinating Board is announced
January 21	Hearing of House Committee on Veterans Affairs, Meridian, Mississippi
January 27–28	DSB Task Force Medical Panel meeting
February 1	Hearing of House Committee on Veterans Affairs on Health Concerns of Persian Gulf Veterans
February 7–8	DSB Task Force CBW Panel meeting
February 22–23	VA Expert Scientific Panel meeting
February 24–25	DSB Task Force Medical Panel meeting
February 28–March 1	IOM Committee meeting and Public Hearing
March 24–25	DSB Task Force meeting
April 20–21	IOM Committee meeting
April 27–29	NIH Technology Workshop: The Persian Gulf Experience and Health
April 29	VA Expert Scientific Panel meeting
May 6	Hearing of Senate Committee on Veterans Affairs: "Is Military Research Hazardous to Veterans' Health?"
May 25	Hearing of Senate Committee on Banking, Housing, and Urban Affairs on Chemical and Biological Warfare
June 9	Hearing of House Committee on Veterans Affairs Subcommittee on Compensation, Pension and Insurance on compensation for Persian Gulf "mystery illness" (H.R. 4386)
June 23	DSB Task Force report released
July 14–16	IOM Committee meeting
July 28–29	VA Expert Scientific Panel meeting
August 5	Hearing of Senate Committee on Veterans Affairs on Reproductive Hazards Associated with Military Service
August 30–September 1	IOM Committee meeting
September 29	Hearing of Senate Armed Services Committee/Force Requirements and Personnel Subcommittee on DoD Response to Persian Gulf Illness

Acronyms

ACGIH — American Conference of Governmental Industrial Hygienists

AChE — anticholinesterases

AFRRI — Armed Forces Radiobiology Research Institute

AR — Army regulation

ARCOM — Army Reserve Command

BaP — benzo-a-pyrene

BIRLS — Beneficiary Identification and Records Locator Subsystem

CARC — chemical agent resistant coating

CBW — chemical and biological warfare

CCEP — Comprehensive Clinical Evaluation Program

CDC — Center for Disease Control and Prevention

CFS — chronic fatigue syndrome

CIA — Central Intelligence Agency

DEET — N, N-diethyl-m-toluamide

DNA — deoxyribonucleic acid

DoD — Department of Defense

DSB — Defense Science Board

DSM-III — Diagnostic and Statistical Manual, 3rd edition

DU — depleted uranium

EPA — Environmental Protection Agency
FDA — Food and Drug Administration
GAO — General Accounting Office
GIS — Geographical Information System
GWS — Gulf War syndrome
HHS — Department of Health and Human Services
HIV — human immunodeficiency virus
IND — investigational new drug
IOM — Institute of Medicine
MCS — multiple chemical sensitivities
MFUA — Medical Follow-up Agency
MRDA — Military Recommended Dietary Allowances
MRE — meal, ready-to-eat
NAS — National Academy of Sciences
NASA — National Aeronautics and Space Administration
NDI — National Death Index
NIH — National Institutes of Health
NOAA — National Oceanographic and Atmospheric Administration
NRC — National Research Council
ODS — Operation Desert Storm
ODS/S — Operation Desert Storm/Desert Shield
PAHs — single and polycyclic aromatic hydrocarbons
PB — pyridostigmine bromide
PG — Persian Gulf
PGW — Persian Gulf War
PL — public law
PTSD — post-traumatic stress disorder
RME — reasonable maximum individual exposure
SCE — sister chromatid exchange
SCUD — Soviet-designed surface-to-surface missile
SWA — Southwest Asia

TLV —	threshold limit value
USAEHA —	U.S. Army Environmental Hygiene Agency
USAMRICD —	U.S. Army Medical Research Institute of Chemical Defense
USAMRIID —	U.S. Army Medical Research Institute of Infectious Diseases
VA —	Department of Veterans Affairs
VAMC —	VA Medical Center
VOC —	volatile organic chemical
WRAIR —	Walter Reed Army Institute of Research